Dos & Don'ts from the book . . .

The *Winner's*

rary

selecting
hairstyles pg. 128

skin care pg. 129

tying a tie pg. 87

tie widths pg. 92

folding
a pocket
square pg. 116

dated lapel
width pg. 65

basic suit
silhouettes pg. 46

basic tailoring
tips pg. 52

do-it-yourself
manicure pg. 135

having trousers
fitted pg. 82

cuffs vs.
no cuffs pg. 80

footwear pg. 107

What Makes
The Style Of
A Winner
So Easy
To Identify?

How Do You
Develop A
Wardrobe That
Really Works
For You?

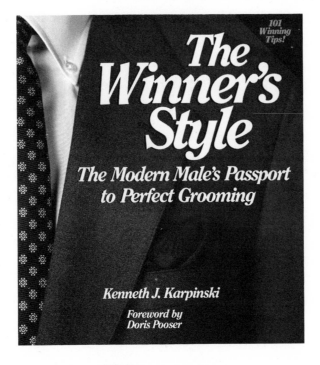

101 Winning Tips!

The
Winner's
Style

The Modern Male's Passport to Perfect Grooming

Kenneth J. Karpinski

**Foreword by
Doris Pooser**

Where Can
You Find
Clothing Styles
Exactly Right
For You?

What Items
Should You
Check Before
You Go
Out The Door?

The Winner's Style

The Modern Male's Passport to Perfect Grooming

Kenneth J. Karpinski

with **Philip Z. Trupp**

ACROPOLIS BOOKS LTD.

WASHINGTON, D.C.

ACROPOLIS BOOKS, LTD.
Alphons J. Hackl, Publisher
Colortone Building, 2400 17th St., N.W.
Washington, D.C. 20009-9964

Printed in the United States of America by
COLORTONE PRESS
Creative Graphics, Inc.
Washington, D.C. 20009-9964

Attention: Schools and Corporations
ACROPOLIS books are available at quantity discounts with bulk purchase for educational, business, or sales promotional use. For information, please write to: SPECIAL SALES DEPARTMENT, ACROPOLIS BOOKS LTD., 2400 17th ST., N.W., WASHINGTON, D.C. 20009

**Are there Acropolis Books you want
but cannot find in your local stores?**
You can get any Acropolis book title in print. Simply send title and retail price, plus $1.00 per copy to cover mailing and handling costs for each book desired. District of Columbia residents add applicable sales tax. Enclose check or money order only, no cash please, to:
  ACROPOLIS BOOKS LTD.,
  2400 17th St., N.W.,
  WASHINGTON, D.C. 20009

Library of Congress Cataloging-in-Publication Data

Karpinski, Kenneth J.,
    The winner's style.

    Includes index.
    1. Men's clothing.   2. Grooming for men.   I. Title.
TT617.K37 1986   646'.32   86-21007
ISBN 0-87491-824-3

Robert Hickey, Art Director
Chris Borges, Designer
Pamela Moore, Artist

Please Note! Every effort has been made to provide accurate color in the color section of this book. Owing to the limitations of the four-color printing process, however, certain discrepancies are inevitable. Therefore, the color samples in this book should be used only as a guideline.

Photos: pages 1, 70—Courtesy of Palm Beach
            pages 12, 16, 20, 42, 54, 138—Courtesy of Country Britches
            pages 34, 62, 84, 106, 114—Courtesy of Cricketeer and Cricketeer Woman
            pages 78, 105, 126, 146—Courtesy of Evan Piccone for Men

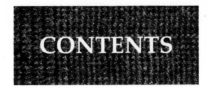

CONTENTS

10 . . . . . Acknowledgments

13 . . . . . Foreword by Doris Pooser

17 . . . . . Introduction

21 . . . . . CHAPTER ONE   Winning Style: A Comparison

Looking Good, 21
Current, Not Trendy, 22
Winners With Style, 23
From East to West, North to South, 27
Corporate Image Checklist, 28

35 . . . . . CHAPTER TWO   Sharpening Your Persona, The Importance of the "Right" Dress

"Boys and Their Toys," 35
Some Case Histories, 37
The 7/38/55 Percent Formula, 39
Little Things Mean a Lot, 41

43 . . . . . CHAPTER THREE   Getting Down to Business: Your Suits and Jackets

Making a Commitment, 43
Fit and Style, 44
Two- Versus Three-Piece Suits, 48
What to Look for When Trying On a Suit, 49
Covering Your American Body with European Clothes, 51
Basic Tailoring Tips, 52

55 . . . . . CHAPTER FOUR **Off-Duty: Leisure Looks**

A "Brief" Report, 55
Hi-Tech Images, 56
The "PA" Principle: Pleasure, Appropriateness, 58
Illusion Dressing, 59
Fine Tuning from More Experts, 60

63 . . . . . CHAPTER FIVE **Homing In On Details**

Women and Other Critical Checkpoints, 63
    Too Small—The Unforgivable Unbuttonable Look, 64
    Piping Around Jacket and Lapel Edges, 64
    Dated Lapel Width, 65
    Fused Chest Piece, 65
    Gangster-Width Pinstripes, 66
    Unmatched Pattern at Seams, 66
    Collar Not Fitting Snugly, 67
    Plastic Buttons, 68
    Gap-osis, 68
    Man-Made Fabrics, 69

71 . . . . . CHAPTER SIX **The Shirt On Your Back**

Banishing the Uglies, 71
    Bloody Collar, 71
    Collar Too Tight, 72
    Frayed Collar, 73
    Fly-Away Collar, 74
    Non-Dress Shirt with a Tie, 74
    Body Too Tight, 75
    See-Through Fabric with T-Shirts, 75
    Contrast Stitching, 77
    Short Sleeves, 77

79 . . . . . CHAPTER SEVEN   One Leg at a Time: Trousers, Cuts, and Cuffs

The Right Stuff, 79
   To Cuff or Not To Cuff, 80
   Pockets Bowing Out, 80
   Horizontal Creases Across Front, 81
   Too Small Waist Size, 81
   What to Look for When Having Trousers Fitted, 82

85 . . . . . CHAPTER EIGHT   The Ties Have It

Tying the Best One On, 85
   Three or More Patterns in One Tie, 86
   Tie Tying Troubles, 87
   Tie Too Short, 88
   Hula Dancers Belong in Hawaii, Not in Your Tie, 89
   Tie Types, 89
   Tie Too Wide or Too Narrow, 92
   Horizontal Crease Across Tie, 92
   Cotton/Wool Knit Tie with a Business Suit, 93
   Tie Longer than Belt Line, 93
   Narrow End Wider than Long End, 94
   Tie Tacks, 94
   Bow Ties: Can They Be Worn for Business?, 95

96 . . . . . CHAPTER NINE   An Introduction to Color

What are Warm and Cool Colors?, 97
Which Seasonal Grouping Do You Fall Into?, 97
Color Planner, Winter, 98
Color Planner, Summer, 99
Color Planner, Autumn, 100
Color Planner, Spring, 101

107 . . . . CHAPTER TEN   Down to the Toes: Shoes and Socks

If the Shoe Fits, 107
How to Buy Shoes, 108
Quality Upkeep, 109
  Polishing Shoes, 109
Footwear Etiquette, 110
  Unpolished Shoes, 110
  Gunboat-Style Shoes, 110
  Dress Shoes and Casual Attire, 111
  Boots with a Suit, 111
  Alligator Nipping at Your Heels, 111
  Skin Showing When Seated, 113
  Black Socks with Everything, 113

115 . . . . CHAPTER ELEVEN   Accessory Etiquette

All the "Little" Things Sure Add Up, 115
  Fat Wallets, 115
  Folding Your Pocket Square, 116
  Pocketful of Pens, 118
  Captain Kangaroo Syndrome, 118
  No "Gorilla-Proof" Briefcases Need Apply, 119
  "Watch" Your Style, 119
  Class Rings with No Class, 120
Better Belt Behavior, 120
  Overly Ornate Buckle, 120
  Brace Yourself!, 121
  White Plastic Belt with Matching Shoes, 121
Eyeglass Frames: Choosing the Right Ones for You, 122
  Selecting Style, Materials, and Color, 124

127 . . . . CHAPTER TWELVE   Your Guide to Perfect Grooming

Projecting Your Best, 127
Hair Today, 128
  Hair Color, 128
  Hair Styles, 129

Hair Texture, 130
Facial Hair, 131
Dandruff, 131
Unbalanced Length—Long Back, No Front, 132
Too Long, 132
Combing Extra-Long Side Hair Over the Top, 133
Poorly Groomed Hands, 134
Do-It-Yourself Manicure, 135
Skin Care, 136

139 . . . . CHAPTER THIRTEEN   Polishing Your Image

Do You Qualify?, 139
Shopping for a Consultant, 140
Using Your Good Instincts, 142
What to Look For, 144
Winning Tips on Consultant Selection, 144

147 . . . . APPENDIX I   Male Maintenance Manual

At Loose Ends?, 147
Sewing on a Button, 148
Missing Buttons, 149
Stain Removal, 150
Food or Perspiration Stains, 150
Removing Stains in Washable Garments, 151
Removing Stains in Nonwashable Garments, 152
Ironing a Shirt, 152
Do-It-Yourself Eyeglass Repairs, 153
Protecting Your Investment, Or How to Decode the
Labels in Your Clothes, 154

156 . . . . APPENDIX II   Winner's Resource Guide

171 . . . . APPENDIX III   Glossary

178 . . . Index

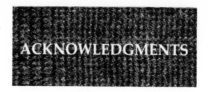

ACKNOWLEDGMENTS

I would like to thank Judy, my wife, best friend, and most enthusiastic supporter, for her patience, love, and invaluable contributions.

At Acropolis, I'd like to acknowledge publisher Al Hackl, who had faith in this project and pushed it through, and John Hackl, Vice-President whose steady support guided it to completion. Thanks also to Val Avedon, who edited out the "bugs" and mentally held my hand; Marg Stanbury, who compiled the glossary, Robert Hickey, Chris Borges, and Pamela Moore, who worked so hard to give *The Winner's Style* a winning look. No book gets far without promotion, and for a good launching I wish to thank Sandy Trupp, Director of Publicity, and Lisa Shenkle, Associate Director; they placed *Style* in the public eye.

For their help and enthusiasm, thanks to B. G. Cox, president of Joseph and Feiss, as well as Sue Smith-Bell, for their expertise and contributions. Van Julian, president of Van Julian Clothing, for his many years of enthusiasm and advice. Sally Frame, president of Talbots, for her warm friendship, support, and her place in Woodstock.

I also wish to gratefully acknowledge the contributions of Harold Nelson, Vice-President and General Manager, Nieman-Marcus, Washington, D.C.; Jon Fultz, of Robin Weir & Co., Inc.; and Greg Mankevich, of the Optical Manufacturers Association, Washington, D.C., as well as Norman Karr, Director of the Men's Fashion Association, New York, N.Y., and Mary Ellen Barone of Palm Beach Clothing, New York, NY.

Thanks to the many consultants: Brenda York, Joyce Jackson, Norma Hoehndorf, Karen Davis, rubye Erikson, Virginia Oakland, Carole Mosbacher, Joanne Hull-Robinson and Diane Neidigk plus countless others whose ideas, experience, and professional advice are quoted throughout.

As is true with any major project, many people were responsible for this book without being a part of the actual process because of what they taught me: Tom McWhirter (for all he taught me about the men's clothing business), Malcolm Katzen (his appreciation of fine quality craftsmanship), Carole Jackson (her love and understanding of color), Dave Mullen and Bob Friedman (who were responsible for my becoming a Men's Clothing Buyer), MaryAnn "Fuzzy" Pownall (for having such a great sense of style), George "Phil" Kelly (who was always there), Larry Gore (for being my menswear mentor).

A special word of thanks goes to Phil Trupp, who was responsible for creating a book we can all be proud of.

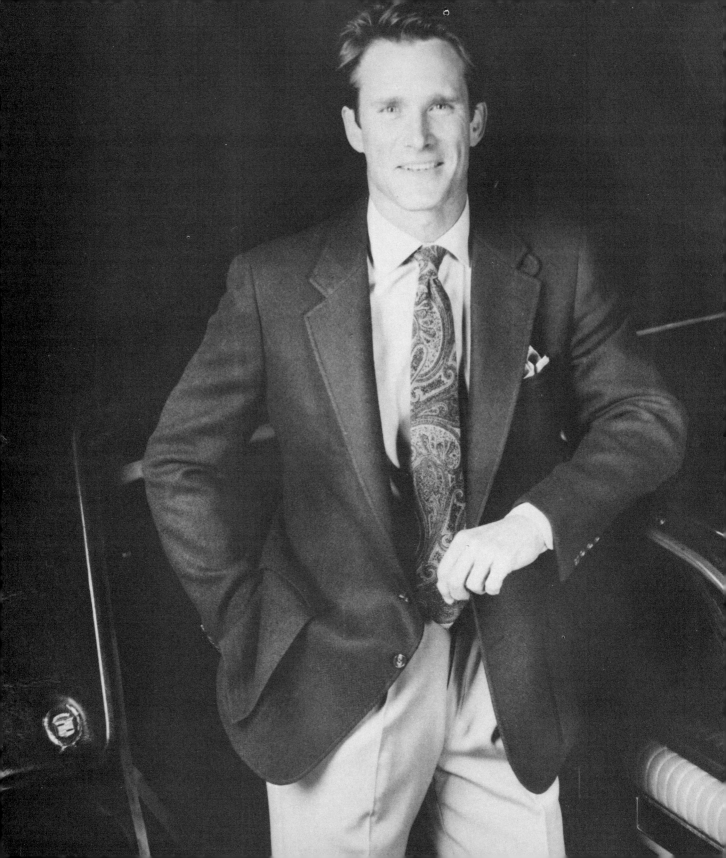

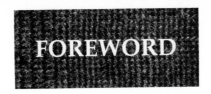

FOREWORD

By Doris Pooser

Author of *Always In Style*

You don't get a second chance to make a good first impression. In the first few moments of meeting someone new—especially in business—goals can be met or missed. Your flow charts, management plans, marketing messages, and product promotions may shine; but they're in your briefcase. To get them out on the conference table with the highest probability of success you must instantly project yourself as someone with poise, confidence, and mature business savvy that adds up to what this book is all about—a *winner's style*!

What is a winner's style?

It's understanding your strong points and knowing how to overcome your weak ones. It means knowing your body line, proportions, and coloring, and wearing the clothes that make the most of these characteristics. It means bringing the best you can be to a world that truly loves a winner.

No two winners are alike, and *The Winner's Style* helps you discover your own individuality. You need to resolve questions you may have about your own body, face, hair, skin tone, and how they affect, in important ways, what you wear and how you wear it. Remember, being a winner isn't a matter of imitation; it's being an original without having to shout about it.

Style and fashion aren't the same things. Fashion changes. Style, because of its individual nature, lasts a lifetime. The well-dressed man must consider both. After all, life is change. Though you can't stop the changes periodically introduced in the mens' clothing industry, you can learn to conservatively adapt them to your special style and enjoy the choices.

How do you develop individual style?

Start by relating style to fashion and the times so that you're appropriately dressed for the occasion. In *The Winner's Style*, Ken Karpinski gives you an insightful look at what's current and acceptable, and what's not. It isn't easy to stay on top of so many developments in a rapidly changing fashion scene; you can get too involved with a busy, rewarding lifestyle to realize that a hair-cut, necktie, or your shirt collar belong back in 1957 with that old Chevy you retired ages ago.

In my *Always In Style* seminars and classes I have helped men and women all over the world define and develop their style and various looks for different occasions. If you know how to select the appropriate shape, fit, and fabric for your clothing, you're on your way to a winner's style, and the rewards it can bring.

These proper looks aren't confined to the office or formal occasions. They carry over to other parts of your life—to a vacation, a game of golf or tennis, and other leisure activities; in these areas, too, you need your own casual look. Today there are wonderful colors, prints, and designs in sweaters, slacks, sport shirts, and shorts for men. Have fun with them!

Now is the ideal time for you to express your personality. The rules are more relaxed and flexible. Choices are infinite. The emphasis is on you—and how well you perfect and use your individuality.

   Whether it's your corporate look, your casual look, or your dressed-up look, everything you wear must be in your personal style. Developing that style is a special challenge that pays substantial dividends. I know you'll find *The Winner's Style* an indispensable book as you embark on a winner's path.

Doris Pooser, Author
Always In Style

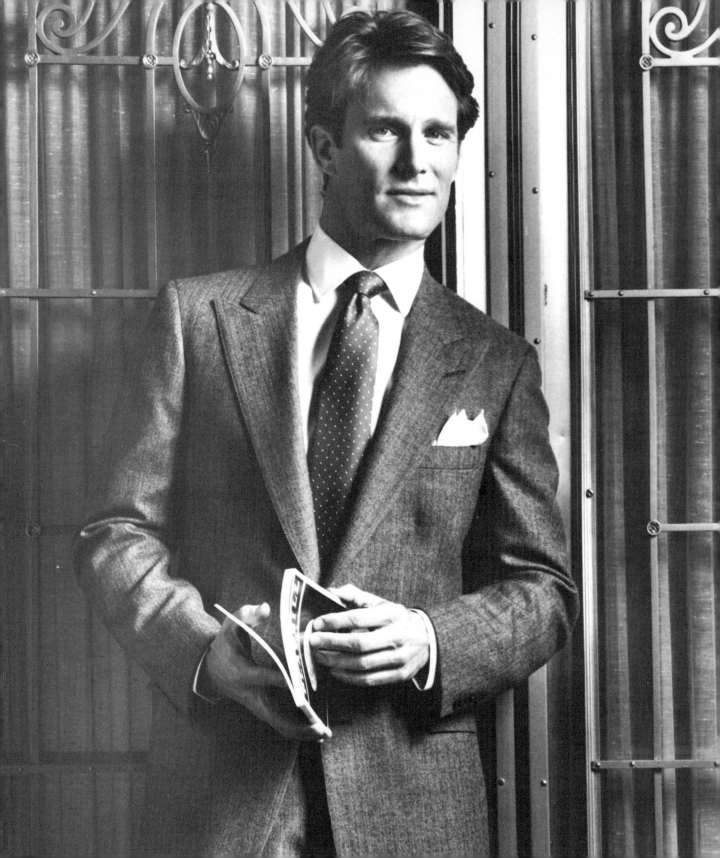

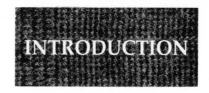

INTRODUCTION

When comedian Billy Crystal tells a guest on his satiric talk show, "Fernando's Hideaway," that, "You look mahvelous!," it isn't just a made-for-television cliché. It's really what most of us want to hear.

Of course, his word "mahvelous" has an abstract ring to it which helps to make it funny. But in the real world, it's a pretty serious business. It means looking great—even if you don't feel so great—and it means looking like a winner, having a "winner's style."

Forget about vanity. Having a winner's style is something we have to work at in a serious, systematic way. And it's certainly worth it. Being a winner can often be its own reward. It means feeling good about yourself. It means getting the most out of life—on the job, at the club, on the playing field, even in love.

There's an old saying in the fashion industry that looking like a winner won't guarantee you a seat on the board of directors, but not looking the part guarantees you won't even get close. Unfortunately, you can't just go out and buy a winner's look, any more than you can fix the Super Bowl or the Heavyweight Championship. You have to go out and earn it, the old-fashioned way.

Earning it involves a number of personal commitments. There is the required investment of time and money, and no small degree of skill and imagination. You need to be in touch with yourself, too; your strengths and weaknesses need to be out on the table where you can see them. You also need to know where you're going and how you hope to get there, and what it is that truly counts for you. You need to develop poise and confidence, a clear vision of what it is about you that you hope to project onto a world that dearly loves a winner. It doesn't hurt to take a lesson in positive thinking from Mohammed Ali, who constantly proclaimed, "I am the greatest!"

Of course you are already on the way to your own championship. Limbo isn't for you. The very fact that you are reading this book reinforces this prediction. It says positive things about you. It says you care about yourself and your appearance in constructive and practical ways; it says you want to project your power points and overcome any not-so-powerful points that may hold you back. You know that like regular exercise and a proper diet, the winner's style is good for you—now and far down the road.

Unlike women, men dress themselves in basic professional "uniforms." For example, in a corporate environment there is the standard two- or three-piece suit (often wool blend), the long-sleeved broadcloth, cotton or cotton-blend shirt, a good conservative necktie, simple leather belt, minimal jewelry, quality watch, serious shoes, and a conservative haircut.

There are, of course, variations to this basic uniform. You'll find them in advertising and other creative fields. Along New York's Madison Avenue, sports jackets of slightly "updated" style are seen. Ties are expressive and colorful; shoes are lighter, and hairstyles are a bit freer.

Physicians often wear sports jackets if they're not in a lab coat; patients don't want to think of their doctors as "businessmen." To get away from a business look they will wear casual ties and comfortable shoes with crepe or rubber soles.

Lawyers and accountants, however, may adopt a "fiscal" or "fiduciary" look: three-piece suits, usually of dark color, quality broadcloth, long-sleeved oxford shirts, conservative silk ties, no nonsense haircuts.

In sales, there are no hard and fast rules of dress. The idea is to dress appropriately for the product and the customer, a concept applied across the board in the 1950s by IBM founder Thomas Watson, Sr., who told his sales force, "Dress the same as your customer." As a salesman, you may keep a change of clothes in the back of your car and make changes, depending on your clients.

All "uniforms" have one thing in common: *specific functional purpose.* They say exactly what the wearer wants them to say. Yet even with the need to adopt the uniform concept, there's some necessary latitude for individual style.

One of the remarkable things about winners is that no two of them ever look exactly alike. They may share certain characteristics, but each is unique, with his own manner and style. (Winners may have to wear "uniforms" at the office, but these uniforms are specifically selected to provide a calm, business-like framework that make their individuality sparkle. It's the man inside that counts, and the winner's style is designed to bring out the best.

In this very special way all of us share in varying degrees the attributes of such successful men as President Reagan, Don Johnson, and "Marvelous" Marvin Hagler, the fiercely elegant Middleweight Champion of the World. They do, on a daily basis, what all of us want to do: assert our independence, our competence, our toughness, our desire to make things go our way. And, like these famous men, we want to be recognized, appreciated, respected, rewarded for being the very best we can be. In reading this book, never lose sight of the inner man or assume that "clothes make the man." They do not! The proper attire is critical when it comes to making the most of your opportunities, to getting your foot in the door when it counts the most. But remember this: the degree of your reward depends on who you are, how good you are at whatever it is you do, and how competently you move through the demanding maze of a competitive society. It doesn't hurt to wear a $1,000 suit and drive a Rolls-Royce Silver Shadow. But eventually you park the Rolls and leave it behind in a garage. The expensive suit may indicate success, but it isn't what closes deals and gets you a nice bonus for a job well done.

Being a winner, with that special "winner's style," always comes back to you. By your appearance you find a means to bring the best of yourself into a world that sees you, touches you, trusts and rewards you. It is a way of putting everything together—a means by which the doors open and allow you to step inside and be the very best you can be.

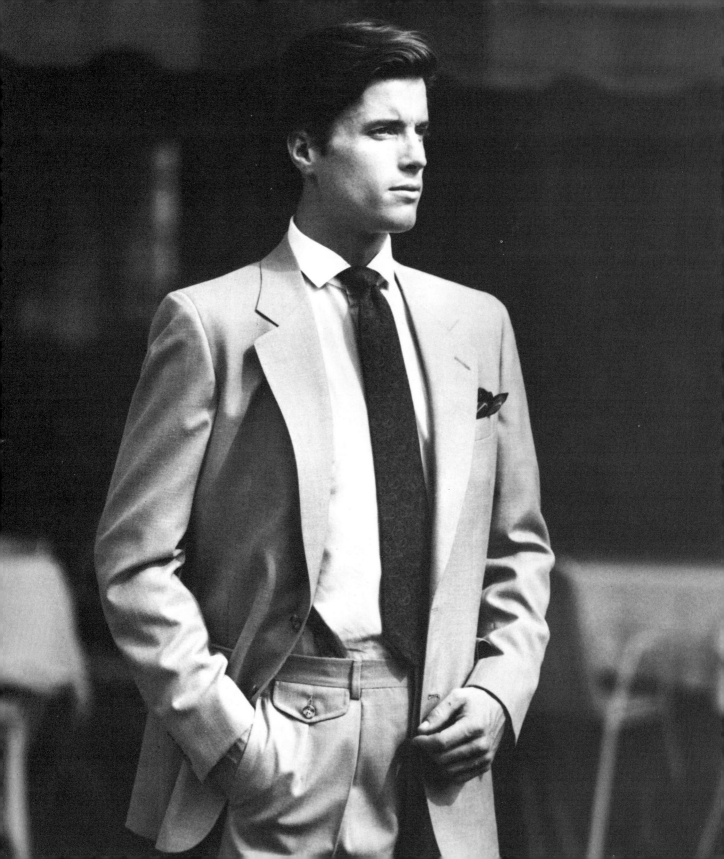

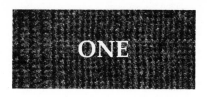

ONE

Winning Style: A Comparison

Looking Good

A tall, slender young man wearing a beautifully tailored double-breasted suit, a blue and white striped shirt and a maroon silk necktie gazes wanly from the cover of the April 14, 1986, edition of *Newsweek* magazine. His identification bracelet is fashionably designed gold; his cufflinks are onyx and pearl. He wears a pearl in his lapel. His watch is obviously expensive and the gold ring on his left hand might have come from a pirate's treasure chest. The magazine's banner headline proclaims: "You're So Vain—Men Are Primping and Preening—And Spending Millions to Look Good."

Inside the magazine, the editors really lay it on. What they perceive to be male vanity, is driven, they say, by the quest to gain "a new sense of self," which includes having your hair permed, pores cleansed, and ears pierced, "to reap the psychic and practical benefits of "looking attractive." And to drive this news home, there is a sidebar story discussing history's greatest fops.

Can all of this be for real?

"It sure is," says Norman Karr, Executive Director of the Mens' Fashion Association, the educational arm of the mens' retailing industry. "It's a function of competition," he says, and it extends from the upper echelons of the corporate world to the locker rooms of the YMCA.

"Affluence is also a part of it," Karr explains. "So you find men doing things they never would have done, say 30 years ago." This includes cosmetic surgery, hair coloring; and, yes, getting your ears pierced. "But you're not going to find a lot of earrings at the board of directors meetings," Karr grins. But there can be no doubt that even at the most conservative levels, style means more than ever.

The message is clear: your competition is working harder to look better, which leaves you little choice but to get in there and slug it out. However, the *Newsweek* story probably overstates the case. Sure, men are more aware of their looks, and looking good obviously makes a big difference. But don't be confused by what the magazine claims is a rush to style "based on casual elegance and polished understatement." For the majority, it's still a matter of conservative elegance, quiet good taste, a style that doesn't stop traffic along Fifth Avenue. Today's male is not Beau Brummell, who wore skin-tight pants, tails, high-collared shirts, polished his boots with champagne and admonished those around him that a perfect gentleman "must change his gloves six times a day."

Indeed, the Twentieth Century executive knows that glitter is a turn-off, foppishness is arcane, and color that looks as if it came from outer space probably belongs there.

Current, Not Trendy

Along with appropriate dress for the occasion comes the need to look current. We're not suggesting high-fashion, trendy, or exaggerated clothing, especially in a corporate environment. It's just not acceptable. But in fields like advertising, television, and public relations, there is more flexibility with colors, designs, fabrics, and patterns. What is important is to keep up with what is new and current, to understand the direction and to reach in this direction slowly according to your personality and the appropriateness of the occasion.

Winners With Style

Fashion and image experts often differ on the ingredients necessary for a man to achieve a truly workable winner's style. After all, experts may have a product or service to sell, blurring their objectivity. Solid, on-the-street advice has its place, to be sure, and is presented here to be constructive and helpful. To kick things off in a practical, everyday way, a group of successful businessmen and women were asked to participate in a "focus group" to decide what wins and what loses in today's business world.

Focus groups are used in business all the time. They generally consist of a half-dozen or more men and women who have experience, directly or indirectly, in a specific field. If a hospital, for example, wants to improve its services, it will call together a group of ex-patients and ask them what they liked or didn't like about the service they received during their stay. In this case, the focus group participants were seasoned business people who are constantly meeting, greeting, and working with clients. Most of them are, to one degree or another, in the public eye and have a thorough understanding of the importance of achieving a winner's style. Taken together, their experience in business adds up to many decades. They have "paid their dues" and speak from first-hand experience. Here are some of our focus group's thoughts:

● **Don Johnson.** This sexy, T-shirted star of the television police thriller "Miami Vice" has no business image whatsoever. He's a sort of "regular guy." In a pinch, his sidekick, Philip Michael Thomas ("Tubbs"), would make a better executive.

●**David Stockman.** President Reagan's former Director of the Office of Management and Budget doesn't live up to his looks. He has style—a practical conservative look—but the man and the style don't add up. His dress makes him look older than his 35 years.

● **George C. Scott.** Like a magician, this actor blinds people to whatever he's wearing. No one notices his suit, his tie; instead, it's his voice, his bearing, that win respect.

- **Thomas A. "Tip" O'Neill.** The Speaker of the U.S. House of Representatives projects a comfortable, confident, wry style. Everything about him bespeaks experience, trust, inside knowledge and a basic honesty. On the other hand, Vice President of the United States, **George Bush**, is preppy, classic and generally perceived as trustworthy, if a little too clean-cut.

- **Anthony Quinn.** This famous screen actor, projects a classic European look, with "earthy" overtones. Whatever he wears, he wears it easily and confidently. Even when he breaks with tradition, his strength of character has a neutralizing affect.

- **President Reagan.** The "Great Communicator" is also perceived as the "Great Image Projector." He knows exactly what to wear and when to wear it. His size 42 suits are of a perfect fabric and cut; his trousers are made with a button-up fly. Soon after his surgery in 1985, he appeared to the press in his California duds—checkered shirt, jeans, boots—all of which said to the American people that their President was not funereal, that he would make it, and to prove it, he was shown at his ranch chopping wood.

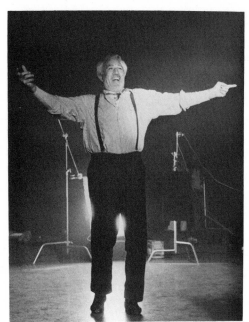

*Anthony Quinn
projects a classic European
look, with "earthy"
overtones. Whatever he
wears, he wears it easily
and confidently.*

- **Johnny Carson:** This star of NBC's "Tonight Show" is seen in the same authentic light as the President. His sports coats accent his low-key, relaxed style. A few years ago, however, when Carson grew a beard, it tended to overwhelm his usual image. Some said it gave him an "evil" cast, others remarked that he looked like an insincere "cowpoke."

- **Tom Brokaw:** This national newscaster is seen as conservative without being stiff, while equally conservative **Ted Koppel,** of ABC's "Nightline" is viewed as a "hairstyle" rather than the professional that he is.

- **Humphrey Bogart:** The late actor is seen as a "dressed-up" Sonny Crockett (the vice cop played by **Don Johnson**), while actor **Warren Beatty** drew unanimous disapproval as "prissy," "cute," or "too sexy to be serious."

- **Caspar Weinberger:** Our Secretary of Defense is, said the group, an excellent dresser, but his grooming? Awful. He's seen as looking "frazzled" and "hassled," and is an excellent example of the notion that a man and his clothing can't be separated. Though Weinberger's suits and shirts and ties are obviously of fine quality and worn with taste, his personal demeanor says "rumpled."

Over and over the group expressed the belief that, in serious business, eye contact precedes attire. Clothing is a big help as long as the standard of quiet good taste is adhered to. Anything that attracts too much attention to itself casts suspicion on a man. And any man who is obviously styling himself after a screen idol or any other public figure is believed to be wishy-washy, someone who has difficulty in making decisions. Another turn-off is a suit that looks so new it "squeaks," or the presence of a flashy watch or pinky ring. Pinky rings go with the Sammy Davis look, the forerunner of the Mr. T. look.

According to the group, a man who hopes to achieve success in business needs confidence before clothing, sincerity above style.

What about leisure looks? Surprisingly, the group applied the same principles used to judge men in a business environment. An example in bad taste: showing up on the tennis court with gold chains around your neck and one of those baffling "sports chronometers" on your wrist. These items are just begging for attention. And this is *not* the way to get it.

This time, the members of the focus group, all of whom participated in some form of non-professional athletics, agreed that "sparkling spiffy sports looks" are the eye-numbing products of today's affluence. The fitness addict, they agreed, often overdoes it. All too often you can tell a real athlete from an amateur by the get-up he's wearing. For example, the late **Jim Fixx,** father of the jogging craze, ran competitively in humble running shorts and a tank top. But the typical part-time pavement pounder goes for a color-coordinated jogging outfit, breathtakingly expensive shoes that resemble Star Wars space ships, a name brand headband, and a chronometer that might have been borrowed from NASA. Thus, the upscale jogger's look says fashion, not sweat.

The golf course, it was decided, is another stage for a technicolor display of the unlikely. **Arnold Palmer** wins world championships in knit shirts and plain slacks. The weekend "duffer" steps onto the tee with a mish-mash of colors and patterns: checkered slacks, striped shirts, orange socks, shoes elaborate enough to be worn by a rock star. Does any of this say "golf"? No way, insisted the focus group. If anything, it suggests a blowout at the clubhouse for those whose scorecards read 175-plus.

The tennis court was viewed as the ultimate conservative arena in which the players must be extra wary of putting on the ritz. If **John McEnroe** and **Jimmy Connors** get away with colorful tops and labels affixed to their shorts, it's okay; they've earned their billboardism, and are paid handsomely for it. But not the weekend "hacker." Fashion forward is strictly out-of-bounds on the court.

One group member was a former golden glover who still occasionally finds time to spar at a local gym. He said professional boxers, such as Middleweight Champion "Marvelous" **Marvin Hagler**, stroll into the locker room in warmup suits and high-top sneakers. Sometimes Hagler wears a jacket with "Marvelous" embroidered on the back. It's a striking contrast to the weekend "canvasback" in "full fluff"—a synthetic warmup outfit that glows in the dark, chic running shoes, and fearsome one-way sun shades. The "full fluff" boxer is perceived as the kind of guy who is likely to sue his opponent for pain and suffering.

Essentially, the group said professional athletes have sweated to earn the right to wear anything they like. But most of us are better off sticking to classic sports outfits that reflect our modest accomplishments. This is to say that if you're not a **Hulk Hogan** or a **Jim McMahon**, forget about being outrageous. And if you can't "float like a butterfly and sting like a bee," your sequined ring trunks will most likely get you floored at the earliest possible moment.

From East to West, North to South

The winner's style, as presented here, is the most universally accepted code of dress. It works no matter where you live or work. Of course there are certain regional differences, but for the most part these are relatively minor. For example, in southern California (in contrast to the northern regions of the state) there is some room for brighter hues, a more relaxed feel, a slightly more expressive style than you are likely to find in the northeast. In Texas, suede jackets and boots are worn, but you had better be a born Texan to make them work for you. In Florida, where weather plays a major role in the way men dress, lighter colors and fabrics are an accepted common sense solution. It would be a mistake, however, to wear Florida apparel for business in Chicago, Seattle, Boston, or New York. Don't try to second-guess regional differences at a distance. Chances are you'll guess wrong. Apply the universal code of quality and quiet good taste no matter where you are, and your dress will never slow you down.

The same thinking also goes, surprisingly, for automobiles, which in the 1980s are said to carry as much personal clout as a perfectly made and fitted suit. The ubiquitous Mercedes, for instance, is perceived as a vehicle best-suited to young women wth time on their hands and money to spend. The Mercedes, today's status machine, seems to cry out to the focus group: sunroof open, cellular phone in hand, and a dozen other status ploys. And the stretch limo says man-of-state or Godfather, while a Porsche sports car belongs to someone who is trying too hard. Cadillacs, according to the group, project the idea of physician, dentist, or middle-aged businessman in search of a little fun.

All of these car critiques appear contrary to our popular beliefs about status and position, and were somewhat surprising. Yet, when added up, the basics come to the surface. The group is saying that anything pretentious doesn't work, that in a subtle way the symbols of wealth, when worn too obviously, emasculate an otherwise strong personality. A man must always have "the common touch," an ease, a sense of trustworthiness, and he must wear his symbols of success in quiet, even modest, fashion.

Corporate Image Checklist

The following checklist, compiled by Brenda York, head of the Academy of Fashion and Image, McLean, Virginia, reflects today's most universally accepted corporate look. Discounting slight regional variations and any eccentricities peculiar to the business you're in, the tips presented here will help you sail smoothly through virtually any corporate environment. It begins at the top and works down to your toes.

Hair style

- Short, conservative cut, styled to complement the shape of your face. See Chapter Twelve for specific shapes and styles.
- Neatly combed, clean, but never stiff or studied.

Facial hair

- If you must have a beard, make sure the hairline stops above your upper lip. If the hair droops down, you'll look sad or bewildered. Of course, neat trim is everything.
- Trim nose hair and any hair growing out of your ears. It isn't a lot of fun, but somebody's got to do it.

Eyeglasses

- Frames should match your skin tones and shape of your face. See Chapter Eleven for specifics.
- No tinted glasses indoors. These have a way of making you look somewhat less than sincere.

- If your nose is long, use a low bridge. For a short nose, have the bridge set higher.
- Make sure the frames don't dominate your face.
- Unless you pilot the company's private jet, avoid aviator frames or any other trendy setting.

Shirts

- For the right fit, make sure you can insert one finger between the collar and your neck. Any more or less and you're in trouble.
- If you have a long neck and face, go for high collars. Short collars work best for short necks and faces. Remember, the collar should flatter the line of your face.
- French cuffs are fine for the office. They add variety. But avoid large cufflinks of any kind.
- Monograms should be subtle. Otherwise, they seem to indicate pretention. If you wear your initials on your shirt front, make sure they match the color of the shirt.
- Cuffs should be approximately one-half-inch below the sleeve of your jacket.
- Avoid short sleeves with a jacket at the office. It just doesn't work.
- Your collar should lie flat against your shirt. If not, you look slightly wilted—or worse.

Jackets

- Go for natural fibers. Try not to wear a suit or jacket two days in a row. These items need to "breathe."
- Be careful to avoid wrinkling across the back or under your collar.
- Good workmanship is paramount.
- Jacket skirt should cover your buttocks.
- The sleeve should end at the top of your wrist. Very small differences look larger than life here.
- Avoid plastic buttons.
- On a sports jacket, metal or leather buttons are okay. They do not, however, work on more formal models.
- Any loose threads? Snip them.
- Steam cleaning is best.

Trousers

- They should have a slight break in front.
- If uncuffed, they should be tapered one-half-inch in the back for the proper look.
- Smooth-fitting pockets. No flapping or bowing.
- How's the seat? If baggy, see your tailor immediately. If tight, see your tailor and your fitness instructor.
- No part of you should be bulging over the waistband. Make it a smooth line all around.
- Well-pressed trousers are a must.
- Pleats should be smooth.
- Suspenders are fine. It's acceptable to wear them if you have belt loops.

Ties

- Don't skimp on a tie. Make it the best you can afford.
- Buy only natural fabrics.
- The color of your shirt and jacket should complement your skin tone.
- Have a little flair. A tie is a personal statement.
- Width should match lapel width. The three-inch tie is standard.
- Tie should end at the top of the belt line.
- The dimple is sexy, some say a little like a woman's cleavage. Still, it's a great finishing touch and perfectly acceptable in the office.
- Tie clips and tie tacks are not as popular as they once were. For the moment, avoid using them.

Belts

- No ornate buckles. It should be simple, classic.
- Should be fine leather or reptile, narrow, and right for the size of the belt loops.
- Buy the best you can afford.
- Colors should be black or brown. The belt must be in good condition.
- Colorful belts are worn only with sports attire.

Pocket Scarfs:

- Complements your tie. It is never identical to it.

Watch

- Make it gold or silver and the best quality you can afford.
- No "beepers," please.
- Roman numerals are classic.
- Thin leather or reptile bands are fine. Metal bands are becoming more acceptable, but leather is still best.

Jewelry

- Confine it to a wedding band, class, or signet ring. In general, the less the better.

Briefcase

- Best is leather, hard or soft.
- If you use aluminum, you had better have a good functional reason for it, such as carrying your Nikon.
- No plastics.
- No combination locks. CIA agents are an exception, of course.
- A briefcase, like your tie, says a lot about you. Buy the best.

Trench Coats

- Ideal length is about two inches below your knee.
- Avoid dark colors. Go for tan or variations thereof.
- Coat should be belted.
- Make it a fine, all-weather coat. It should travel well.

Socks

- Should match slacks or shoes.
- Black, blue, and gray are best for business.
- Covers calf. No skin showing.
- Argyles are for casual wear only.

Shoes

- The best quality you can afford.
- Keep them polished. Every day isn't unreasonable.
- Laced shoes and slip-ons are acceptable. Slip-ons are more stylized, laced shoes more sober.

- Loafers with tassels are fine with a sport coat.
- Wingtips are on the way out; they're considered too awkward. Thin soles are preferred.
- Dark color. Anything bright catches the eye and detracts.
- White shoes for casual wear only, and best with white suits.
- Avoid wearing the same shoes two days in a row.

"Wanna know
if a guy is well-dressed?

Look down"

George Frazier
columnist, *Boston Globe*

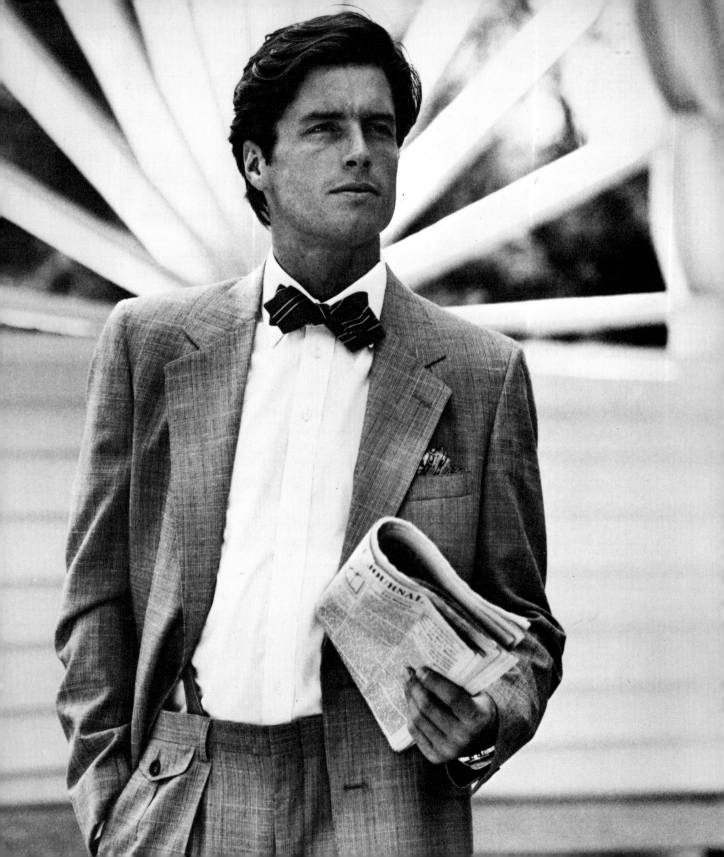

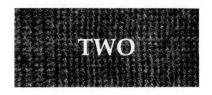

TWO

Sharpening Your Persona: Importance of the "Right" Dress

"Boys and Their Toys"

There's a common misconception that men don't change very much as they grow older, hence the chestnut: "The difference between men and boys is the price of their toys!"

Indeed, this saying has a nice settled ring to it, a comfortable old shoe aura. If only it were true. The truth is that men do change, sometimes in radical ways. From boyhood to CEO, they must continually adjust to these changes and update their persona. If they fail to do so they are stuck in a rut, and this is a prelude to disaster in every facet of their lives.

The psychology textbooks are filled with the ups and downs of male "passages," their changing needs for love, praise, recognition, and money. There are hundreds of ways to accommodate these passages, but the one we are going to deal with here is the way in which men influence the way others relate to them, how the world "out there" sees them.

Long gone are the days of the "me generation" and slogans such as, "You can't judge a book by its cover." Publishing houses have long since proven that covers may not tell you what's inside a book, but the cover is the reason that we pick up one or another off the rack. Until it is picked up, no sale is made.

Men are in the same position. And, to overcome resistance, they use the one tool that is at their disposal and completely under their personal control: *outward appearance.* This book is designed to help you use this "cover" to its greatest advantage.

Of course there are changes in "cover," adjustments dictated by dozens of factors ranging from the physical to the professional. As we grow older or simply move through the various stages of our career, we need to adapt our outward appearance to project who and what we are. A major object of these changes is to present to the world the image of being a person who deserves to get the greatest rewards.

While it is true we are all individuals, a recent informal poll about sought-after goals revealed that most of these desires fall into a fairly small number of categories.

Some Case Histories

 DAN R. (A Case Study)

Dan R. can be referred to as a dentist to the stars. He has a very successful practice, an active social life rubbing shoulders with the rich and famous, and a fulfilling family life. When asked whether he considers a person's appearance very important, he replied, "When I was in dental school I thought it mattered not a bit, but a seemingly minor event changed my mind about that. My wife and I were invited to a barbeque. The invitation read: Dress: informal. The event was being given by a corporate president on a big farm. When we arrived along with our good friends, we observed the "farm" filled with several hundred guests. Every man on the grounds was wearing a sport jacket, many with neckties. My best friend and I had on short-sleeved knit shirts and slacks (mine happened to be jeans). Ben, my friend, went to the back of his car, opened the trunk and pulled out a navy blazer, put it on and disappeared into the crowd. I felt like a fish out of water all evening. One woman even asked me to bring out another bag of ice, assuming I was with the catering service. It was one of the most uncomfortable times I can recall, and though I had anticipated making a lot of high-level contacts, I ended up spending 3 hours behind a bush with my wife, watching everyone else have a grand time.

BILL B.   (A Case Study)

Bill B. is a senior partner of an oil and gas investment firm. He is a very meticulous person in all aspects of his life and after an incident a few years ago believes that most people, despite what they say, do judge a "book" by its cover. Here's what happened. One of his "rookies" (a salesman still in his first year with the firm), came into his office very upset. He thought he had made his first big sale. For weeks he had been selling this heavy hitter client (one who can write a check drawn on his personal account for $150,000) on a drilling program the company was raising funds for. He would call and write, but the morning he went in person to the client's office to pick up the check, he found the client distant and somewhat preoccupied. After only a couple of minutes came the news, "I've changed my mind; I've decided not to invest in your program." He stood up and showed the young salesman out.

In an effort to save the sale, Bill picked up the phone and dialed the near-client's private line to see what had happened. After a brief introduction, Bill asked if the client would explain his sudden change of mind.

"Have you ever taken a look at him and would you hand him $150,000 of your money?"

Bill then took his first close look at the rookie. He confessed he could see exactly what the client was talking about. The rookie really was a mess. His eyeglasses had tape holding the frame together; his tie was food-stained; he looked rumpled and his shoes were in need of a shine. In short, he didn't project a credible or professional image. Bill brought a currently popular self-help book into the office the next day and told the rookie to "close the door to your office and don't come out until you've finished it." Then he showed him a check in the amount of the commission he would have earned had the sale been closed—nearly $12,000.

"This is how important the way you look is," Bill said. "Fix yourself up."

Five days later, Bill and the rookie came out of the formerly reluctant client's office with a check in the amount of $200,000. Hard evidence of the importance of a man's appearance.

The 7/38/55 Percent Formula

 GARY S. (A Case Study)

Gary S., an executive in his late thirties, believes he learned the importance of how a man dresses dates back to the days he spent in prep school. The fellows with whom he prepped came from a wide range of backgrounds, both culturally and financially. The one element they all had in common was their school blazer.

"Once you put on your blazer you became an equal. People gave you the benefit of the doubt, got to know you as an individual." As he grew older, serving in the U.S. Air Force and then in the business world as a management trainee, he observed that people immediately formed opinions about those with whom they came in contact. This opinion was based on nothing more than the other person's appearance. He also said that at least a dozen times in recent years he has heard other senior executives say, "they just don't look right" when reviewing prospective employees. The job candidates may be equally qualified but simply don't know how to put themselves together—dressing- and grooming-wise—in a business environment, so they lose out. After all, these guys will be representing the company to the outside world! To show you how important **Gary S.** thinks the subject of looking the part is, in his office is a paperweight inscribed with the following, credited to professor Albert Mehrabian, "To develop trust and believability, 7% is what you say, 38% is how you say it, and 55% is how you look."

CASEY G.   (A Case Study)

"I never used to think much about it," recalled **Casey G.,** a financial planning advisor, "but I've changed my mind. I worked with an expert who evaluated and cleaned out my closet and then went shopping for replacements. I can now say I enjoy going shopping and I'm considerably more confident that I project a successful, prosperous image to my clients. In my business that's important. Let's put it this way," he says. "Maybe it's just a coincidence, but this year I will earn more money than ever before in my life and my wife loves hearing other women's compliments on the way I look when we attend parties. One thing I am sure of, though, is I can concentrate on the business at hand when meeting a new client and don't have to think about my image. I know it's first-rate."

 ## CARTER H.   (A Case Study)

Carter H. is Vice President of Operations of a rapidly growing consumer products company with offices around the world. He just finished moving the company's headquarters to new, enlarged facilities. He requested proposals from several large waste removal firms. He reviewed three firms that seemed reasonably priced and set up appointments to meet with their representatives. The first two were just short of what he was looking for and so he decided to wait and see what No. 3 had to offer. As it turned out, No. 3 had everything he was hoping for in terms of service and financial arrangements. But when the rep came in, he couldn't believe his eyes.

"The guy was a walking disaster," says Carter. "He really looked like he had just posed for a "don't let this happen to you" poster. From the top of his unkempt hair to the bottom of his well-worn heels, this fellow was a mess."

Carter has a fairly simple code of business dealings: "I only do business with people and companies I can respect and who respect me, as well."

Carter proceeded to tell the rep that while Company 3's proposal was superior to the others, he could not consider doing business with his firm. The prospect of having this man in his office on a fairly regular basis seemed unthinkable and if this is representative of the waste removal company as a whole then they must be pretty shoddy, too. And yet, the bid was good, very good. Under the pretense of scheduling a second appointment, Carter called the sales manager of Company 3. In the course of the phone call he brought up the subject of appearance in a not-too-subtle way.

Three days later, the Company 3 salesman was back, beautifully dressed and impeccably groomed. Carter couldn't believe his eyes. He signed the contract on the spot; a deal that was worth nearly $10,000 to the young man, who has since gone from near the back of the pack to the No. 2 salesman in the company.

Little Things Mean a Lot

 ### PAT A. (A Case Study)

Pat A. is a nationally known sales trainer who works with virtually a "who's who" in American business. He is regarded as a master of telephone selling techniques. He is quick to point out that, more often than not, agreement on the phone is only half the job no matter how well it is handled.

Most people want to meet the people with whom they do business and the way you present yourself will greatly influence how others perceive your opinion of yourself and your company's attention to detail. What we are seeing is that more and bigger companies are paying attention to the way their sales and marketing staffs look when working with their accounts. Actually, it's the little things like shoes, neckties, and briefcases that are helping create the overall professional image that people are comfortable doing business with.

These case histories make the point with which we began this chapter: *men change!* In these cases, the changes led to getting what they wanted. By placing a fine gloss on their appearance they learned that getting what they want and need is often a matter of looking as though they deserve it. In short, think like a winner, act like a winner, take the winner's style and a lot of the formerly "impossible" obstacles to success will vanish.

CHARLIES'
SERVED DAILY 11:30 am

e DAY
omato SALAD
SON
ALSON

SALAD
SALAD
LAD
IÇOISE

GER
BURGER

LET of SOLE
ALLOPS
SCAMPI
the DAY
STEAK
EAK
E RIBS
CALF'S LIV
HALF CHIC
VIENNO
SIRLOIN
BROIL
the DAY
SALAD
BOARD

8.50

THREE

Getting Down to Business: Your Suits and Jackets

Making a Commitment

Buying a suit is a little like getting married. You have to shop around—very carefully. You have to try this one and that one, sweat and puff and scrutinize until you find one that *may* work well with who and what you are. Having gotten that far you want to make a "commitment" because any further indecision seems futile. So you boldly move ahead where all other men have moved before, sometimes successfully, sometimes to your regret. You start to cull your choices. You walk around with the suit, sit in it, check out every angle while anonymous salesmen nod and smile and occasionally offer reasonable advice. "It's you, sir," they say as you squint before the three-way mirror. The tone of voice sounds oddly like your fiancé's roommate, the matchmaker. All the while you realize that the salesman, no matter how well-meaning, isn't invested sufficiently to call the shots for you. It's up to you.

In the end, you've gone as far as you can go with the ifs, ands, and buts, and you hear yourself saying, "I'll take this one."

The salesman grins. "Good choice, sir."

It had better be, cause it's going to cost you and it's got to be worth it. On the way home you pray you've done the right thing, and by the time you close the door behind you you're determined that suit *will* work—no matter what, for better or for worse.

There is no way that I know of to make buying a suit a waltz. It's a tough job and you've just got to do it. Unlimited funds—the idea that it's only money—won't help, either. Expensive mistakes are still mistakes, and poor choices always still add up to a loss.

Fit and Style

Norman Karr, of the Men's Fashion Association, feels that too much is made of body types and the kinds of suits that are supposed to be right for them. No matter if you're tall, short, thin, muscular, stocky, or corpulent, most of the suits on the market today will work for you if the fit is right, and you have chosen the correct silhouette to begin with.

There is, for example, an old myth that says portly men should never wear double-breasted suits. "It's not so," Karr explains. "Lee Iacocca wears double-breasteds all the time, and he's no small guy. The tailoring is perfect, and that's a lot of the battle."

The variety of suits on the market these days can be mind-boggling, but basically there are four kinds (with variations):

1. The "Natural Shoulder" Suit. Known as the "sack suit" when it was developed at the turn of the century, it is typical of American style and tailoring. It has a square front, unpadded shoulders, rolled lapels, and pocket flaps. President Theodore Roosevelt wore this model, and it became the rage among those who wanted to emmulate the Rough Rider's bold, broad-chested look. The first models had three or four buttons on the jacket; the three-button model won out because the lapels could be longer, giving the wearer a trim appearance. The jacket was slightly snugged at the waist and hips. It took a Democrat to change

these details. President Kennedy was a sworn two-button man, and Brooks Brothers, sensing a trend, came out with a twin-button version—this in the face of protests by some of Brooks' tailors and designers. It remains today as the traditional "ample cut" suit of classic American design.

2. The European Cut. This suit has padded shoulders and fits snuggly at the waist and hips. It is often seen with side vents on the jacket. The trousers have slightly flaired cuffs. There are two and three button models. Its intent in design is to produce a slim, trim look by staying away from the traditional American full cut.

3. The "Updated Traditional American," cut is styled to reflect fashion trends. Depending on what's in, it may have side vents or a center vent. The shoulders may be padded and the jacket shaped to conform to fashion flows. The easiest way to look at this silhouette is to think of it as a mirror of current fashion that offers a certain amount of flair.

4. The "Athletic" Cut. This silhouette is becoming more popular, particularly on the west coast and to a lesser degree in the New York City area. This model has a drop from chest to waist of between eight and ten inches. Cut with larger shoulders and thighs, it is perfect for the swimmer or body builder who in the past had to have extensive alterations to obtain a proper fit.

None of these designs is cast in stone, however. Changes are constantly being introduced. What's important to keep in mind is that trendiness has no place in business. In the board rooms across America you are most likely to find the classic traditional Brooks Brothers style, and reasonable facsimilies. This is where appropriateness comes into play. The uniform has to fit the occasion, which is to say that you can wear any suit in its proper place.

A suit's silhouette and how it conforms to your body shape is more important than fabric, color, pattern or details despite what fashion experts have been espousing. If the silhouette is wrong nothing, including alteration, is going to save you. So get this part right and all the rest is a plus.

Natural Shoulder	*Modified American*	*European*	*Athletic Cut*
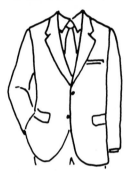	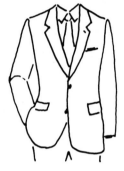	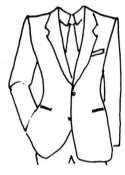	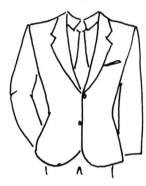

Chest and waist measurement are approximately the same. Under 5'10" the shape would be considered square/sturdy; over 5'10", rectangular/built like a brick; if waist is larger than both chest and hips rounded is the only description. If waist and hips are both larger than the chest a pear shape.

The ideal size for this silhouette is a body measuring a six-seven inch drop, the difference between your chest and waist measurements (if you measure your chest to be 40 inches and your waist is 34 inches you have a 6 inch drop). This body has enough "natural" shaping to be flattered by the nipped in waist and only slightly padded shoulders of the updated model.

Particularly suited for thinner men in professions that permit a bit more fashion expression (retailing, advertising). The average American male's body with its broader shoulders and fuller chest often is not comfortable in this cut. Because of its sleekness of line and details (long, narrow, peaked lapels; ventless, slash pockets; lower seated, tighter fitting pants) it is often favored by females. This style accounts for only 10% of sales nationally.

Due to the health consciousness of many of today's men, the three main silhouettes were not able to fit properly an ever growing segment of the population. The body builder or swimmer with his large powerful shoulders and chest and small waist, often with large muscular thighs. To fit this guy the athletic suit was designed. It has an 8" to 10" drop from chest to waist, fuller cut sleeve head (where the sleeve attaches to the body) and more fabric through the thigh for comfort. If you have, for example, a 46 inch chest and a 36 inch waist then the athletic cut suit or jacket may be perfect for you.

"Fit and appropriateness are the two unshakeable rules," says Norman Karr. When it comes to the business of fitting suits to differently shaped bodies, he believes that fabric and fabric pattern count for more than anything else—after fit, of course.

A portly or stocky man should stay away from plaids, horizontal designs, heavy fabrics, such as tweed. These make him look broader. His best bets are wool blends, pin stripes, solid colors.

Very thin men do well with heavier fabrics and high visibility checks and other patterns. The patterns fill them out.

As for muscular men, they, too, have to be cautious about patterns. Too much pattern in a suit can exaggerate their natural lines and make them appear ungainly. The well-tailored double-breasted models, however, look great. Sylvester Stallone made this point between his movies, "Rocky I" and "Rocky III." In the first film he wore badly fitting suits, but later, when he won the title, he dressed in double-breasted and single-breasted models that made him look like a millionaire, which is exactly what he had become in Rocky's third incarnation. Once again, perfect tailoring paid off.

See Appendix II for specific men's clothing designers.

Color, of course, is another matter and will be discussed later, beginning on page 96. For now, it is enough to say that blue and gray suits are the accepted corporate colors, and are often considered "power suits"—strong, bold, yet quietly elegant. The darker tones give the wearer a firm presence without calling undue attention to any single element of the design.

Light and mid-tone colors can't be ruled out entirely. American style allows a certain amount of freedom, but the basic corporate wardrobe contains the standard blues and grays, almost as if the members of any corporate body were born to wear them.

Two- Versus Three-Piece Suits

There are two basic questions men have raised at my seminars:

1. Are three-piece suits out?

Basically, the answer is no. Three-piece suits have been the uniform for decades. Men have accepted this uniform and the inherit lack of freedom in expressing themselves associated with it. What it really means when you look in the stores and see more suits consisting of two pieces than three, is that it's an economic decision on the part of the designer, not a fashion statement of what's in or out. As the price of a well-constructed suit climbed beyond the $200 mark, stores became more and more anxious that the buying public would not accept this higher-priced merchandise. With $275-$300 pricetags, stores envisioned a dramatic decrease in sales. By eliminating the vest, and encouraging two-piece suit sales, they were able to stay at or around the $200 price range, which was much more acceptable to the general public. The bottom line? It is AOK to go for that three-piece suit; don't give up the right to decide for yourself if that is the suit that will help you find your winner's style.

2. Are fully lined suits an ultimate sign of high quality?

For years, salesmen have been telling customers that "full-lined" was an indication of quality. In the beginning, there was some truth to that equation, but as the garment industry grew into the "off the rack" business as we know it today, things changed. Initially, winter garments were made with very fine heavyweight piece goods and had a full lining to add an additional layer of protection from the cold. It also helped the jacket slide on and off easily, and to lay smoothly on the shoulders. As a rule, summer suits were wool-blends of lighter weight. Since the extra protection wasn't needed, only half-linings were sewn in. So you can see that it was logical, if not entirely correct, to equate quality with linings.

As the business became more "mass-market," manufacturers found that not putting a full lining in actually caused them a great deal of extra work. The seams had to be sewn very evenly, trimmed carefully, and then pressed flat in order to look respectable when examined. By putting in a full lining they could hide compromised construction. So while a full lining doesn't automatically mean a suit is first-rate, it doesn't mean shoddy, either.

What to Look for When Trying on a Suit

No matter how beautifully the color of a suit complements your personal coloring, or how fabulous the "hand" of the fabric, you can't achieve an overall good look if the fit of the garment isn't correct.

You don't need to become a tailor to ensure your next suit fits you properly. Most good stores employ competent people to measure and fit you. But you still need to understand what you are looking at when you gaze into that three-way mirror so you can maintain your half of the conversation with the man with the tape measure around his neck (or pins in his mouth).

Here is an easy to follow set of guidelines to allow you to feel confident while being fitted:

- The collar of the jacket should hug the back of your neck. If there is any space, it must be corrected. Should you see a horizontal bubble of fabric just below the collar between your shoulder blades, do not be overly concerned. It can be eliminated by lowering the collar. A fairly routine alteration.
- The back of the jacket should fall smoothly and follow the curve of your back with no vertical creases. Depending on the fabric and pattern the center seam can be let out or taken in.
- Make certain the jacket bottom (skirt) covers your rear end. Too short a jacket will look awful, too long a jacket will lengthen the torso unattractively, and make you look like you are wearing a "zoot suit."
- The correct sleeve length is the point where the hand meets the wrist. Simple. Be aware of two things when having this measured: 1) have both arms measured; most people have one longer than the other. 2) You should be wearing the long-sleeved shirt you will normally wear when being fitted. One-half-inch of shirt cuff (sometimes referred to as linen) should show beneath the jacket sleeve.

- The waist of the jacket should conform to your own waistline. Only minor adjustments can be made here. If it hugs you too tightly or droops over you like a potato sack, you need a different cut of suit.
- Your shoulders should not bulge out past the sleeve head (that is the point where the sleeve is attached to the jacket shoulder); what you should see is a smooth line, from the shoulder all the way down the sleeve.
- The vent or vents in back should not pull open when standing erect. Of course this does not apply to the ventless styles since there is no vent to pull open. When considering a ventless model, be very honest with yourself. You must be fairly slim in the hips and not overendowed in the rear. Whatever model you are considering—ventless, single-vent, or double-vented (also referred to as side-vented)—your trouser seat should not be seen.
- The front of the jacket should lie flat across your chest. When buttoned, the jacket lapels should lie smoothly, with no bowing out. If there is more than one finger's space between the lapel and your chest, the next size or another model should be tried on.
- Make sure that your trouser creases are clearly visible from the bottom portion of the side pocket opening all the way down. If you see any horizontal lines at the waist, thigh, or knee areas, the pant legs are too tight and should be let out.
- Don't forget your belt. The fit of the waist band is every bit as important as the cuff. When trying on a pair of trousers adjust your belt to see how it feels.
- Most suits are mass-produced, particularly the ready to wear varieties. It's important to check the alignment of the buttons. Also, check to see if the bottom of the jacket lines up when you button it.
- If you're active in your suits or have a job in which you move around a lot, do the same thing at the clothier's. Tailors will usually fit you as a more-or-less stationary type. So move, bend, twist. Make sure the suit does the same, comfortably.
- Most of today's suits don't have "top stitching"—zig-zag stitching on the outside which is, in fact, the designer's "signature." You'll find top stitching on European-made suits. It can be removed safely without the suit falling apart. It's best, of course, to have the tailor handle it.

- If you're purchasing a three-piece suit and the vest has an adjustable belt at the back, button the vest and tighten the belt so that it feels comfortable. Then sit down a few times and check the feel. Remember, if you commit to a three-piece suit you will be removing the jacket but not the vest. Make absolutely sure the vest is comfortable and non-constricting when seated.

- If you carry your wallet in your inside breast pocket, bring it with you to the store and place it in the pocket when being fitted. This allows the tailor to adjust for the extra room that will be needed to accommodate it. Do the same for the pants if you keep your wallet in your back pocket.

- At all stages of the fitting—as well as in the selection process—keep in mind Beau Brummell's advice. He said if a person turns to observe your dress, your clothes are "too new, too tight, or too fashionable."

Covering Your American Body with European Clothes

As with everything else, the rules for determining how the European sizing system translates into American body types seem to be made to be broken, so your safest bet is the most obvious: try it on first. The following guides, though, should help put you in the ballpark:

Throughout the continent you can use the following with a fair degree of confidence:

Necktie Sizes *(inches/centimeters)*

US	14 in.	14½	15	15½	16	16½	17	17½	18
Europe	36 cm	37	38	39	40	41	42	43	44

Sweaters/Sportswear

	Small		Medium		Large	
US	38	40	42	44	46	48
Great Britain	38	40	42	44	46	48
France	44	44/46	48/50	50/52	54	
Italy	48	50	52	54		

Shoes

US	7	7½	8	8½	9	9½	10	10½	11	11½
Britain	5½	6	6½	7	7½	8	8½	9	9½	10
Continental	40½	41	41½	42	42½	43	44	44½	45	45½

Basic Tailoring Tips

When it comes to having their suits fitted, many men look upon their tailors with awe. Like a chat with the family physician, men often assume the tailor can cure just about anything, given a list of symptoms. Unfortunately, it doesn't work that way.

Quality clothiers try to employ competent, experienced tailors, but they're busy people, working under deadline pressure, and there is a tendency to work to "type" rather than your specific—and sometimes peculiar—needs. On a hectic day it's all too easy to miss the finer points. It's up to you to guide the tailor through a fitting and ensure that what you're buying is exactly right for you.

The following is a list of critical details to check with a tailor. Some of these points may seem obvious. Bring them up anyway. At today's prices, it's better to be safe than sorry.

- The break of a pant leg at the bottom depends on the height of the heel of your shoe. When being fitted, be sure you bring your business shoes with you—not your sneakers.
- When it comes to hemming the pant, specify how you want it done. If you want a cuff, say so. If you don't, the tailor will almost automatically hem a cuffless style.
- Ask the tailor if you can expect any significant amount of shrinkage in the dry cleaning process. Today's fabrics have allowed for all sorts of cleaning processes, but play it safe and ask anyway.
- Wear a long-sleeved shirt when being fitted for a jacket. It's the only sure way to insure proper sleeve length for your coat. The right fit allows for one-quarter- to one-half-inch of shirt cuff to show below the jacket sleeve.
- Don't stand completely erect. You don't stand that way to begin with and you're not being fitted for a uniform, so why have your suit fitted like one. Stand as though you're in your office talking to a client in person, leading a meeting, conducting an interview. Visualize where you will be with that suit on, and with whom. Remember, you're not the cowardly lion walking into a store wanting to have a suit fitted as if you were really the tinman, and you certainly don't want to walk away with the suit that makes you look like the scarecrow.
- Treat the tailor you feel most comfortable with as your doctor; understand that he's not out to make you look bad; he's out to make you look every bit as good, if not better, than you think you look and are. Let him in on the type of business environment you're in, or the occasion when you plan most to be in a suit.

Most retail stores carry not only extensive lines of suits, but in most cases carry shirts, ties, belts, shoes, socks . . . all the little items which go *with the suit* you are purchasing. Allow the retailer to suggest a certain shirt and tie combination or a tie and pocket square combination. Use your own best judgment after getting to know the retailer, but in most cases, if you handle things in this manner, you're apt to minimize the stress involved in pulling it all together, or waking your wife or roommate for a second opinion before departing for work.

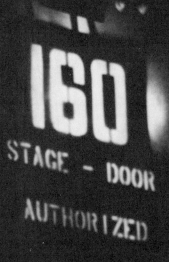

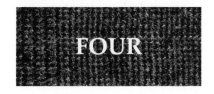

FOUR

Off-Duty:
Leisure Looks

A "Brief" Report

These days, the male passion for style goes well beyond the boardroom. More than ever, it seems, men are striving to look great to the world outside—and, in particular, they want to appeal to the opposite sex.

While some may argue that there's nothing new in this age-old drama of boy meets girl, professional image and color consultants claim that men are playing their roles with renewed intensity and flair.

"If you doubt it, I suggest you take a close look at men's underwear," says Brenda York, an internationally known consultant, whose Academy of Fashion and Image, in McLean, Virginia, concentrates on the burgeoning male image-consciousness.

Just a few years ago, she says, baggy boxer shorts were as common as black socks. But no more.

"These days, you see sexy bikinis in vivid colors," she explains with perfect professional sincerity. "And, believe me, age is no barrier when it comes to who buys and wears them."

She conjures up a rather fun image:

"Think about Lee Iacocca. Could it be that underneath those perfecty tailored business suits of his he's wearing red, white, and blue hip-huggers? I wouldn't be a bit surprised."

What it adds up to, she says, is that men, in seeking the attention of women, are tired of being "boring." They enjoy seeing their women in sexy briefs, so why not a little pizzazz for the guys? "It's a way of saying, 'Hey, look at me. I can be sexy, too.' "

Mike Dickerson's company, College Concepts, Inc., produces boxer shorts emblazoned with fifty different college logos as well as most N.F.L. teams emblems. He sees the trend toward fun underwear this way: "First, people are looking to be a little irreverent, not run of the mill, to display a bit of uniqueness. Second, they enjoy being part of a group and being able to be identified with it, though not in a boring, stuffy way."

Hi-Tech Images

While men have plenty of information available to them on dressing for the office—if nothing else, they can observe what their more successful colleagues are wearing—in the area of casual wear the guidelines are vague, at best.

This is rapidly changing, however, and there is now a computer program developed by Joyce Jackson, of Ultimate Image of Burke, Virginia, which matches a man's body features to different styles of clothing and produces a customized and prioritized listing of "Personally Identified Clothing Choices," known as PICC. The program can generate as many as 59 million combinations. An individual reading costs as little as $45.

"PICC takes the concepts of image and color one step farther," says Norma Hoehndorf, a Beauty for All Seasons executive director working out of Virginia. "With the computer, we can really zero-in on what's best for you—and it really goes from head to toe."

Beauty for All Seasons, headquartered in Idaho Falls, Idaho, has 14,000 consultants world-wide, and a division called Man for All Seasons. Given the vast network, PICC is bound to make a strong case for computerized styling, especially in the leisure area.

Can PICC help when it comes to attractiveness?

"Oh, definitely," says Hoehndorf. "All the time we see good-looking men wearing things that don't work for them. The program can find the best styles for particular body and face shapes, and it goes into tremendous detail."

Of course, there's no absolute of sexiness, she explains, and much depends on what makes a man feel good about his appearance. And, just as men have personal opinions about attractiveness in women, so women have their own views about what makes a man attractive. It's probably the most subjective judgment anyone can make.

Hoehndorf's organization has made a stab at it, however, and has come up with four male "looks"—rustic, conservative, aristocratic, adventurous. These categories combine clothing styles and personalities. Here's how it breaks down:

- **Rustic:** This is the strong, silent, outdoorsy man. He is basically friendly, approachable, athletic, and unpretentious. Rustics are supposed to look good in easy-going styles, such as tweed jackets.
- **Conservative:** This category includes a great many men, that in a way represent the official size and weight of American males. The conservative is level-headed, trustworthy, correct, professional, but he cares about making the best of what nature has offered. He looks good in single-breasted blazers, muted plaids, Izod-styled sports shirts.
- **Aristocratic:** These men are supposed to have "classy" tastes. They are very self-assured, authoritative; they give off an unmistakable air of formality. They wear things like a six-button peaked lapel blazer. They tend to dark colors, but they combine "rich" combinations, such as green and blue.
- **Adventurous:** These men are "daring," and they are similar to Rustics, except that they wear more fashion colors and styles. The main thing about them, physically, is a striking set of features. They are free-thinking, devil-may-care, up-to-date. They are also "Romeos."

All of these men, says Hoehndorf, are going in for "fun clothes," and the sorts of attire that give them a feeling of confidence.

"No matter what type a man is," she says, "most are after a trim, updated leisure style. It's hard to describe exactly. It's sort of what you might imagine Secret Service men look like on the weekend—a casual but planned appearance, with a little dash thrown in."

The essential elements of sexiness for males (besides bikini briefs!) include proportionately styled clothing, the proper hairstyle, perfect grooming, a reasonably fit body, and an air of confidence.

There is yet another element, Hoehndorf explains.

"The average (female) man-watcher looks at men from behind. I know it's kind of a cliche, but it's true. Women look at 'buns'—a man's *derriere.* It tells them if a guy's in shape. Along with that is his walk. If he shuffles or is kind of slew-footed, that indicates that maybe he's a loser. But if he's got a lift to his walk, it means self-assurance, a winner. It's not very scientific—certainly not on a level with the PICC computer model—but it is a part of female judgment about sexiness."

The "PA" Principle: Pleasure, Appropriateness

One of the major concerns when it comes to casual clothing is the individual's perception of what constitutes "personal style," says Karen Davis, head of Color Concepts, Alexandria, Virginia. "Men get kind of lost here, because a definition involves so many elements."

Lifestyle is a major factor, along with body, color, and the kind of clothes a man feels good in. And what a man does with his after-office off-hours is a primary consideration, too. Does he spend his leisure hours at art galleries, movies? Does he go for long walks, engage in direct activity or go in for spectator sports?

"I'm not talking about athletic clothing," Davis explains. "You wear specific functional clothing for sports." She says there is a gray area between the office and the playing field, and it's here that men need to make careful judgments about the styles that do the most for them.

"I tell my clients to go for the pleasure principle," Davis says. "Leisure clothes should make you feel good. After that, they should be appropriate for the occasion."

Illusion Dressing

Karen Davis is an advocate of what she calls "illusion dressing." Essentially, the concept focuses on a man's physical assets and liabilities; the emphasizing of the former, and the minimizing of the latter. She uses her athletic, six-foot, eight-inch husband as an example. He wears a size 48 jacket and has a narrow waist and hips.

"Because he's a big guy, his jacket lapels are medium-sized rather than narrow, and he wears pleated trousers to add a little bulk at the bottom. His belt is chosen to match his shirt rather than his pants, which shortens his very long torso. He has a long neck, so he wears long collars." The overall affect, Davis says, is to make the most of his stronger characteristics.

Davis insists that it's difficult, at best, to define exact male body types; most, she says, are a mixture, a puzzle which "illusion" dressing aims to solve in the most flattering way possible. The idea, she explains, is based on "scale"— bone structure, height, and width-wise proportions.

"You can take a football player and a basketball player and find many of the same characteristics in both," Davis says. "That's where the concept of scale comes in. Basically, it takes into account bone structure, height, and weight. Unfortunately, men don't often think of these features. They think of style, or fashion, and that can really throw you off."

For example, "Style A" may fit a tall man or a short man. That's fine, as far as it goes. But "Style A" may look good only on one or the other, not both.

"In casual wear," Davis says, "scale is everything, almost. What flatters you is what's best—not what's most fashionable or in. To me, getting that formula right is a big part of looking sexy and appealing to women."

She claims she can tell regional origins just by looking at a man's casual attire. The Davis formula sees the following:

- **Midwesterners:** They look relaxed, basic. Conservative, but not fussy. They tend to be understated and hardly ever display a fashion-forward look.
- **Easterners:** "In a word, 'preppy,' " she says. "It's the L.L. Bean Look."
- **Southerners:** They're colorful, casual, very relaxed in manner and appearance.
- **West Coast:** Stylish. Fashion-forward. They wear lots of accessories. "In a word, they have 'flair.' "

But Davis always comes back to appropriateness as a common denominator of what makes a man most attractive.

"Think of President Reagan dressed like Don Johnson (star of "Miami Vice"). Now that's not sexy. But think of Don Johnson as Reagan, and that is sexy because it's appropriate dress for the Oval Office." She also points to former President Jimmy Carter, who tried to popularize informality in the White House—with utterly dismal results. "Carter looked foolish dressing like a peanut farmer and going on national television."

"The main thing is that a man should feel good about himself," she says. "Again, it's pleasure and appropriateness that's the bottom line."

Fine Tuning from More Experts

Ms. rubye Erikson of Color Me Beautiful in Minneapolis, Minnesota, says: "Things to watch out for, for young and old alike, are wearing the inappropriate shoe for the occasion, such as too casual of a shoe with a dress-up outfit, or a business-style shoe with jeans or worse yet, shorts." She adds, "Heavy men should avoid tightly knit polo-style shirts," for obvious reasons!

According to Virginia Oakland of Virginia Oakland and Associates of St. Louis, Missouri, and an In Style consultant, "Men have never been more concerned with their total image. Today's man realizes that image doesn't stop after he leaves the office. He has to look sharp, act sharp, dress sharp, and be presentable to the public at all times. Well-coordinated image-dress for a man's casual, social, and sports life is considered as important a business as business dress itself."

Carole Mosbacher, president of Carole Mosbacher and Associates of Kansas City, has been trained by both Color Me Beautiful and Always In Style. She says, "Men can have many looks, not just one. Business, sporty, and romantic, depending on what is appropriate for the occasion. Finding the right line and color is imperative to be believable in many looks."

And Bobbie Jean Thompson, of Image Reflections for Body and Wardrobe, in Charlottesville, Virginia, feels that the principle of optical illusion must be understood by a man as well as a woman, in order to achieve one's optimum appearance. A man will have to spend a lot of time and energy to catch up to the knowledge that a female has on fabrics, texture, color, body proportion, line and design, in order to create his own style. She continues, "It is not a reflection on ones masculinity or intelligence to seek professional help for body proportion and wardrobe planning."

This is an opinion shared by Joanne Hull Robinson, head of a firm called One on One Fashion Consulting which operates out of Woodward's Department Stores in Vancouver, Canada. Men of all walks of life comprise nearly 30 percent of her firm's clients. She believes casual wear is becoming more and more important and offers this piece of advice to all of her male clients: "I call it 'Third-Piece Dressing,' which means: Don't put on a shirt and slacks and think you are ready to go out. Always bring a third piece into play and pull it all together. A sweater, jacket, or vest will give you a much more finished look. Even a woven belt or watchband which coordinates with the colors of the pants or shirt will do wonders."

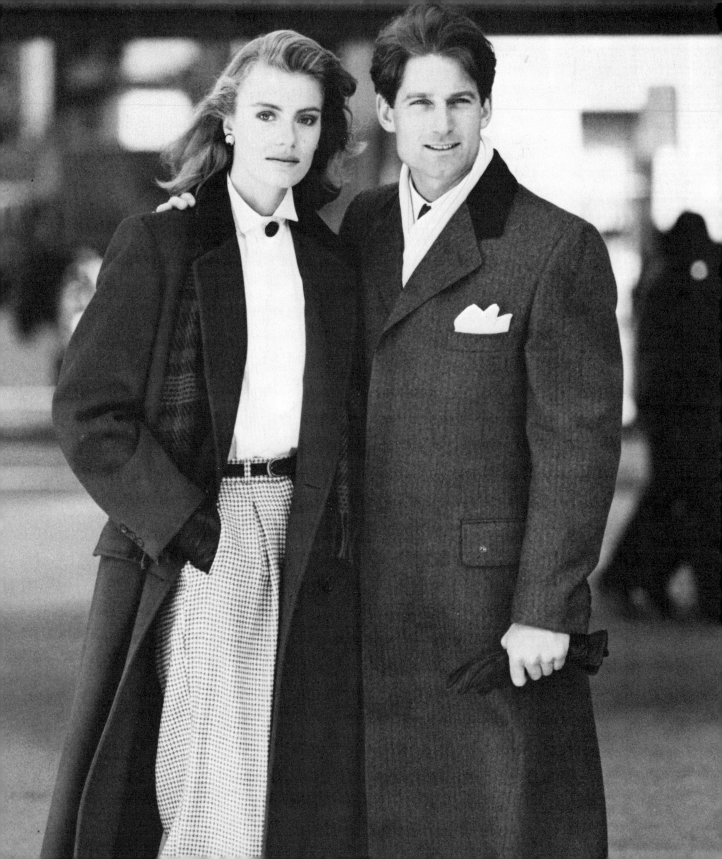

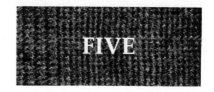

FIVE

Homing In On Details

Women and Other Critical Checkpoints

Now that you've learned the basics, it's time to focus on those make-it-or-break-it details of fit, fabric, and style. You probably won't want to memorize them, so to give yourself every advantage it might be a good idea to reread this book before your next shopping excursion.

Before I go on, however, I want to mention the importance of a woman's eye in this rather tricky business. The woman (or women) in your life has a keen sense of what works in a man's wardrobe. After all, your mother was probably the first person to dress you, and subsequent females, including wives, have continued the line of succession. While it's important to develop your own eye and sense of taste, the woman's "feel" in these matters can be more than a little helpful. It may be a good idea, too, to lend this book to the women in your life. Their critical appraisal can really pay off and save you a lot of unnecessary aggravation.

The professional fashion or image consultant is an invaluable aide. Women in this growing industry tell IBM, Chase Manhattan Bank, Burroughs, and other huge corporations how to do it. They are paid for their experience in what works and what won't—and they get amazing results. When considering a consultant for your own purposes (a subject I'll discuss at length later on) remember that when these high-powered women talk, even E.F. Hutton listens!

Here, now, are the critical checkpoints:

Too Small—The Unforgivable Unbuttonable Look

All too often your weight, or should I say your overweight, is the reason for looking poorly dressed. If you button your suit jacket or sport coat and the lapels do not lay flat against your chest, but bow out away from you, then your jacket is probably too small. If you can't button it at all, then it most certainly is time to move up and buy a larger size. Don't try to convince yourself that you're going to lose weight and in 30 days this 40 Regular will fit perfectly. All too often you won't lose the weight. Better to buy the 41 or 42 Regular; and, if you do trim down, have it taken in—or reward yourself by hanging it in your closet to remind you how great you look when you're trim!

Piping Around Jacket and Lapel Edges

I cannot think of a single reason for anyone to own a jacket with contrasting color around its edges or lapels. A little research suggests that the origin for this fashion detail was the colored stripes or bands on ancient Roman garments, which were used to denote rank. But it isn't acceptable in today's business environment. To be perfectly honest, it doesn't work in many social circles, either. It says cheap.

The one exception is a western-style sport coat of wool or wool-blend, edged in a very subtle shade of genuine leather, complimenting rather than contrasting the color of the jacket. You need to be careful not to abuse this exception. While it is a look much more at home at a casual outdoor affair, some parts of the country do allow it to be worn in business settings that are not too formal.

Dated Lapel Width

Several years ago a group of men's clothing manufacturers decided to give men a reason to shop for suits more often. They reasoned that if they adjusted the width of the lapel every year or so, men would have to replace their clothing more often or else look badly dressed.

The effort was such an unmitigated disaster, and you can rest assured that the width of men's suit lapels won't vary too much from the 3–3½ inches now seen on most men's clothing.

Of course, as with any rule, there are exceptions. A few designers are working in slightly narrower lapels. Accessorized with the correctly proportioned shirt and tie, it is a very nice look.

A fairly safe rule of thumb for any situation is to wear a lapel width that is very close to half the distance from the inside of the lapel to the shoulder. You can't go wrong.

Fused Chest Piece

For a jacket or suit coat to hold its shape, it must have what is called a "chest piece." Generally this is made of coarse fabric and fits between the outer fabric and the lining. It is held in place in one of two ways. First, it can be fused, which means glued. This is the less expensive method, which has several drawbacks. It produces a very stiff front panel that doesn't conform to your body's movements. Also, except for the highest quality, the glue has a tendency to melt at high temperatures. So after a couple of trips to the dry cleaners, the front of your jacket will sprout small blisters of fabric. Currently, there is no way of repairing this damage.

Second, a manufacturer can sew in the chest piece. This is most often done by hand and is therefore a rather expensive process. This produces what is referred to as a "floating chest piece." The advantage to you is a very soft, springy jacket front that keeps its shape, moves when you do, and won't be hurt by frequent dry cleanings.

The bottom line: avoid having your jacket stand up before you do.

Gangster-Width Pinstripes

Men's suits exist in solid colors, patterns such as herring bone, tic weave, plaids, and pinstripes. By far the preferred uniform of American businessmen is the pinstripes. While it is very difficult to go wrong with many of the various types of stripes, it can be done.

Basic pinstripes differ because they are either formed by a series of beads or by a chain link pattern, or they have different space between the stripes. These spaces range from 1/16-inch to as wide as 1 inch and are generally a safe bet. Candy stripes are a fairly recent trend and use a colored thread such as blue, red, or yellow instead of white to form the pin stripe. As long as the effect is subtle, "candies" can liven up your wardrobe, yet remain businesslike. Chalk stripes are also found in quality clothing. The effect is similar to the line that is created by a tailor's chalk on the fabric, and for the most part, they are very subdued and sophisticated. However, you can get into trouble if the chalk stripe is too wide or in too much contrast with the suit color.

The rule is, if you can see that it is a stripe from across the room, be careful! The width, contrast, or spacing may be too extreme for business use.

Unmatched Pattern at Seams

One of the most time-consuming and expensive features that can be very easily seen by the average shopper is how carefully the pattern (whether stripe, herringbone, or plaid) is matched at the seams. The finest products will have a virtual mirror image at any point that two pieces of fabric are sewn together.

If you were only to check a few of the most important points, check the back seam, the lapels, and the collar. From a distance this may not be a very noticeable point; but, up close, it is obvious.

The simple reason that more manufacturers don't do it is expense. To lay out all the pieces of a pattern by hand is a very time-consuming task that naturally adds to the labor cost. In addition, it means a waste of a great deal of fabric. At between $10 and $20 per yard for fine piece goods, this can add up.

Many mass-produced lines use a computer to lay out patterns so that virtually no fabric is wasted. That only helps the maker; it's no advantage to you unless the savings are passed on. I'm afraid we have not reached that phase yet.

Collar Not Fitting Snugly

Nothing can ruin the look of a suit or sport coat faster than an ill-fitting collar. If you put on your jacket and the collar doesn't lay flat against your shirt collar, exposing about ½-inch of shirt, your jacket's collar needs to be adjusted. While this isn't as obvious as a too-small garment that can't be buttoned, it does identify the wearer as someone who doesn't know how the article of clothing should fit. Either that, or they buy their clothing at an establishment that has salespeople or tailors who don't know what they are doing.

There's really no reason to allow this fit problem to persist as it's a very easy alteration for a qualified tailor. A precaution: since lower quality clothes often do not have a hand set collar, it's a bit more difficult for a tailor to reattach the collar perfectly.

The opposite problem is a "bubble" of fabric just below the collar of the jacket and is usually centered on the back seam. It can be avoided and once again, any qualified tailor can correct it quickly and economically.

If a person turns to observe your dress,
you are not well-dressed;
instead,
your clothes are either too new,
too tight, or too fashionable.

Beau Brummell

Plastic Buttons

Most of the buttons on a man's suit or sport coat are not there to work. They are for decorative or historical reasons only.

One particularly fine suitmaker is a fellow named Warren K. Cook. The firm that bears his name produces one of the better makes of suits available in Canada with limited distribution in the U.S. He has replaced the three or four buttons on the jacket sleeve with what is referred to as the "Cook Shield." This is an enameled "button" with the family crest emblazoned on it. To my knowledge it is unique.

People tend to use plastic to replace the bone buttons found on the finest of suits. I think this is an economical measure not in the customer's best interest as plastic buttons tend to break more often than bone.

Gap-osis

Gap-osis is the condition that exists when a man's vest does not come down far enough to cover his belt line, and a line of shirt fabric shows through between the vest and pants. The most prevalent cause of gap-osis: extra poundage that seeks out the upper body. The vest is meant to be snug fitting, but not *that* snug.

Now, don't try and kid yourself. Don't stand in front of the mirror, suck in your gut, pull up your chest, pull down your vest, pull up your pants, and proudly declare that all is well. Stand relaxed, with the bottom button upon (some hefty monarch is said to have decreed this and you know how we are about following orders). If any of your shirt is peeking out, be assured that it is going to get worse after sitting and getting up a few times. There is no way to camouflage this situation, and the best advice is don't wear the vest until or unless it fits properly. It conveys all the wrong things about you. It doesn't matter if a suit costs you $800, "gap-osis" strikes rich and not-so-rich alike. Young as well as old are its victims.

Man-Made Fabrics

The polyester of today is vastly improved from the original.

Due to advances in technology, most of the disadvantages that existed, such as stretching, bagging, and snagging, were minimized or eliminated altogether once manufacturers realized polyester could be spun, patterned, and woven to resemble wool. It also can be woven together with natural fibers to create a soft, resilient, and practical blend.

When added to an equal or greater number of natural fibers (wool or cotton) it creates a garment that stays neat and crisp looking and has a degree of breathability (though not as much as a 100 percent natural fabric). It is actually superior in terms of upkeep and keeping its shape throughout a long plane flight or steamy day in the city.

One area where man-made fibers still lack is the way they take colors in the dying process. With most basic suit and sport coat colors this doesn't seem to be a problem, but be careful if you are looking at a "fashion color."

---

*Boots and shoes are the greatest trouble
in my life.
Everything else one can turn and turn
about, and make old look like new; but there's
no coaxing boots and shoes to look better
than they are.*

George Eliott
Amos Barton

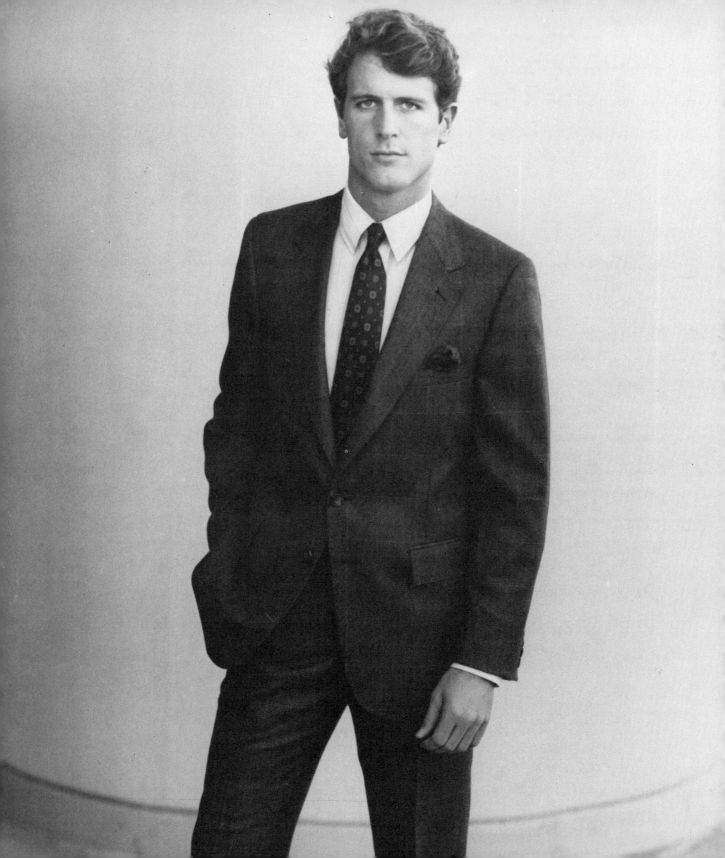

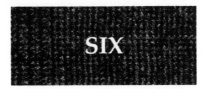

SIX

The Shirt On Your Back

Banishing the Uglies

We have already zeroed in on many common errors—those little "uglies"— that men are prone to inflict upon themselves. It can be pretty hard to swallow the "uglies" all at once, but now that you're generally familiar with them, we'll serve them to you in palatable doses, providing you with the antidotes that make this section especially important.

Take heed; along the way we may prick some sensibilities and put pressure on longstanding prejudices and opinions. But that's the way it is with change, and achieving the perfect winner's look means excising the "uglies" to the backwaters, where they belong.

We promise to make this as painless as we know how to, and like medicine you take for a cold, keep in mind that it doesn't have to taste good to be good for you. If you can take it you're going to be a lot better off. You'll feel better, look great, and open doors that may have been closed in the past.

Bloody Collar

Just picture this scene: You have traveled halfway across the country to give a major presentation that may affect your next promotion or raise. You awaken promptly at six o'clock in order to have plenty of time before your eight o'clock meeting. You shower, shave, and order room service.

As you flip up your shirt collar to insert your tie neatly underneath you fail to notice that the minor nick on your neck has begun to bleed ever so slightly since you removed the piece of tissue that seemed to help stop the bleeding.

You now look as though you are a failed suicide attempt. Everyone who you come in contact with will notice—much to the detriment of your presentation and hoped for promotion, raise, or sale.

While razors, blades, and lathers have improved to nearly eliminate the chance of nicks and cuts, don't forget a time-honored remedy to be packed in your toiletry kit—the styptic pencil. This little lifesaver contains as its active ingredient aluminum sulphate, and can dry up a cut in seconds. If it's too late for the styptic pencil to come to the rescue, be prepared for emergencies.

Always tuck an extra shirt and tie away in your bag just in case. If the bloodied garment is white, check with the hotel desk clerk for a drop or two of Wite-Out,™ the typewriter correcting fluid, for a cover-up. If all else fails, acknowledge your nick up front, move on, and don't worry about it.

It's also wise to have an extra shirt tucked away in a desk drawer at the office—collisions with the coffee machine have been known to happen!

Collar Too Tight

Some of today's best dressed, most fastidious men allow this to happen. Even those with custom-made shirts may do it, though the custom experts generally try to save them from themselves at the initial fitting.

Here is how to avoid this "ugly": When buttoned, your collar should be loose enough to insert one finger between your neck and collar comfortably. If you find you can't do this, have your neck re-measured. You'll likely need a larger collar size.

Aside from slowly strangling yourself, which is bad enough, if your collar is too small, your tie cannot sit properly underneath it, and the points of your shirt will not lay or roll properly if it's a button-down.

Attempts to make do with a too-small collar are usually unsuccessful. They include: moving the top button over, enlarging the buttonhole with a razor, even attaching a button to an elasticized ring that fits over the original button. The latter idea is the least offensive, and is better than turning your collar button into a possible lethal projectile every time you clear your throat.

Frayed Collar

Few areas receive as much abuse as the top of your collar at the back of your neck. It's a case of out-of-sight, out-of-mind.

When a shirt is laundered and starched, it is done so flat. Then it's pressed flat, folded over, and pressed again.

When we put the shirt on we flip up the collar, slip a tie around the neck, and fold the collar over this. Then, the hair on the back of the neck scrapes away at this already weakened area (did you know that hair has the tensile strength of aluminum when dry?) for week after week.

Other than having an adequate supply of shirts to allow for a little relief between wearings, there is not much you can do to prevent wear unless you buy custom-made shirts. With custom-made shirts, you can ask to have the collar replaced if it starts to go before the rest of the shirt. If custom-made is not for you, be sure you inspect your shirt before you put it on and toss it in the rag pile if it's starting to give out!

Don't think that if you let your hair grow down over your collar no one will notice. They *will*. Turning the collar one-quarter-inch usually ends up displaying the tie in back . . . *not* an acceptable alternative.

Collar Types

button-down   regular   rounded   spread   pinned

Fly-Away Collar

When you wear a standard spread collar, the points should rest lightly on your shirt. Two reasons for this not happening are:

- The tie is either too wide or too heavy. When tied, it produces a knot that is too large to fit comfortably under the collar points.

  Be careful when combining a tie that has been an old friend with a new shirt. Collar point lengths change from time to time, so take this into consideration. If you want to try a different collar style, treat yourself to a new tie, too. In many stores, the shirt and tie buyer is the same person and will work closely with you to ensure a proper fit.

- The tie is missing collar stays. Stays are the plastic strips that fit inside the thin groove sewn into the underside of a collar point. Most cleaners remove these before pressing to avoid accidentally melting them. They may neglect replacing them and leave you in the lurch if you've packed for a trip without double-checking. Buy plastic replacements (very inexpensive) and always have a couple stowed away in your travel kit.

Brass collar stays also work very well and come in several sizes. Unlike plastic you can't trim them with scissors to fit, but you'll be a lot more careful to remove them when you send your shirts to be laundered.

An early mentor of mine at Bloomingdales once told me of a time he was away from home and found that he was missing one of his two collar stays. Ever resourceful, he trimmed the edge of a recently expired credit card to fit. It worked, and he swears he'll still cut his cards in half when they expire but he won't throw the halves away.

Non-Dress Shirt with a Tie

A flannel shirt with a knit or woven tie is very much at home with a Harris® tweed sport coat but it is not considered proper in most business settings.

A fine cotton Tartan plaid shirt with a coordinated linen woven or cotton knit tie is super for informal weekend wear; as is the knit polo-type shirt with 3-button front placket worn with a properly informal tie.

If you are working your way into the boardroom, avoid:
- aviator shirts with epaulets (unless, of course, you are a pilot);
- front pockets with flaps and buttons;
- any type of contrasting stitching or trim;
- a pattern that falls outside of the generally accepted stripes, tattersall plaids, pinstripes, pencil stripes, university stripes or—for the more adventurous—a bold stripe body with white collar and cuffs.

Body Too Tight

Ready-made shirts are available in approximately one-half-inch increments of collar and sleeve measurements, the bodies are cut in proportion.

The type of fit varies by manufacturer and even by different lines of the same maker. Generally speaking, there are three "cuts" of shirt:
- fitted, a very trim silhouette;
- traditional, often referred to as a gentlemen's cut, fuller across the chest and not as nipped in at the waist; and,
- full, exemplified best I think by the shirts made by Brooks Brothers.

Full shirts are very comfortable, but many men find them a bit too roomy. One co-worker told me he never wears his Brooks Brothers shirt in Chicago, fearing a rogue gust of wind will send him skyward.

If your buttons pull, your front placket doesn't lay flat against your stomach, or horizontal creases appear across your chest, it may not mean that you're too fat. Rather, you may be trying to wear a cut that is inappropriate for your body type.

See-Through Fabric with T-Shirts

While wearing an undershirt keeps its wearer comfortable and protects expensive outer garments from unsightly perspiration stains, it should be appreciated, and never seen.

Your choice of undershirt styles is limited to crewneck, vee-neck, and tank top-singlet. We definitely don't want to discuss long underwear here, but if you're wearing see-through fabric, be sure to wear an undershirt with it.

While seeing the outline of your undershirt is better than revealing chest hairs, or the lack thereof, you should try to match the style to the occasion. The crew neck is the best for most business situations. However, when your plans call for you to wear a shirt that is open at the collar, consider switching to a vee-neck. This way you get all the benefits without sharing your underwear with the world.

Most military branches and some civilian occupations have uniforms that are open at the neck. Army regulations require a green or olive drab crew neck T-shirt with open neck fatigues or battle dress uniforms. If you fall into this category, have a few crew necks for when you "dress up," but try to stick to the vees for day-in-and-day-out use. Other than its light weight, I have found no major advantage, or proper use, for the tank top unless you work outside and remove your outer shirt regularly.

On clean-shirt day
he went abroad,
and paid visits.

Samuel Johnson
Boswell's Life of Dr. Johnson

Contrast Stitching

If you own a shirt with contrast stitching, do not wear it with a tie. Ever! (This means a shirt where the thread that connects the cuff to the sleeve, pocket to the body, and runs around the collar and down the front placket is of a different color than the body of the garment.) Reserve these shirts for your leisure outfits—perfect for a Texas Bar-B-Que, for instance.

Short Sleeves

In some areas of the country during the summer months, a short-sleeved dress shirt is perfectly acceptable. "Guayaberas," for instance, are beautiful and very practical formal shirts, worn in South America. However, give some North American men a sartorial inch and they will do their very best to take a mile. Just because it's "OK" where you live, don't expect others to automatically accept this form of business dress when you travel. They won't.

In most large urban areas the work place is air conditioned, as are most cars and homes. There simply is no real reason to wear short sleeves. If the heat bothers you, try a cotton or a good cotton-blend shirt with long sleeves. You'll be surprised at how comfortable they can be.

If you need to keep the wrist area clear of fabric for work-related reasons, fold the cuff of your long sleeved shirt under into the sleeve; don't roll it up on the outside. Folding it under will keep it up and still present a neat appearance.

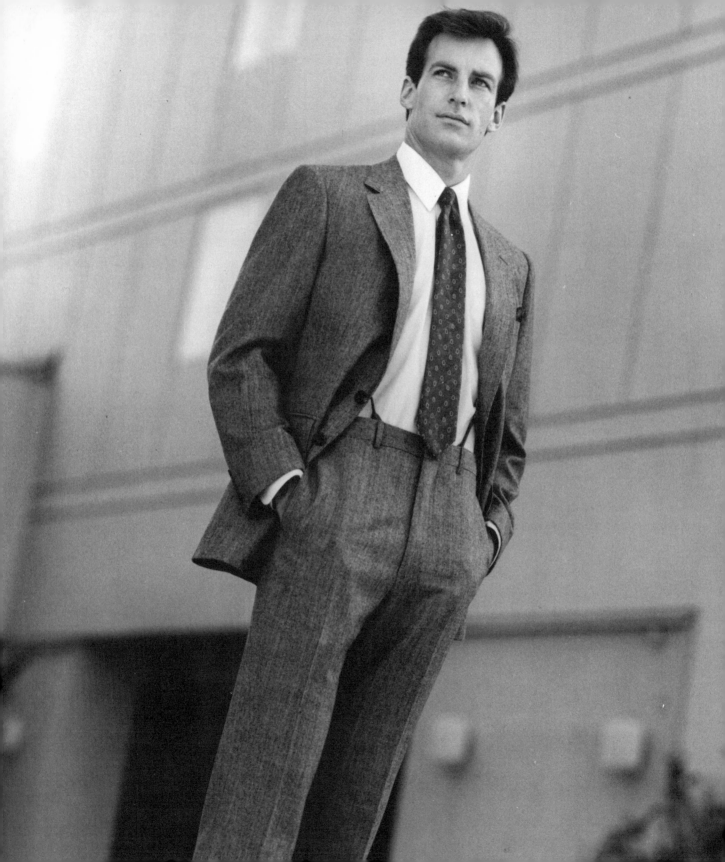

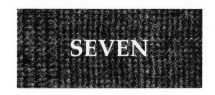

SEVEN

One Leg at a Time: Trousers, Cuts, and Cuffs

The Right Stuff

"Few items of apparel are more critical to the way a man *feels*—and looks–than his trousers." Everything else may be perfect, but if your waistband is compressing you like a Victorian bone corset, if your thighs are numb from loss of circulation, if you're hiking them up or pulling them down, if your seat is threatening to erupt, it's definitely time for a change.

If you should doubt the importance of trousers, remember that we grow in and out of them faster than anything else we wear. The constant battle against the forces of gravity can never be won completely, and so hardly a year passes when we are not reminded by Mother Nature that it's, alas, time for another adjustment. Though the fitness fans among us aren't confronted as often, they too must eventually deal with expanding tape measurements.

You need the right trousers for the right look. Actually, the best fit is probably one that lets you forget about your trousers entirely. *Easy* is the operative word. After all, you've got enough to worry about in your busy, competitive life without having to "sweat it"—literally!

When it comes to pants, the facts really aren't too tough to tackle. A few simple rules will get you by comfortably for the rest of your life.

To Cuff or Not To Cuff

Beyond some common sense guidelines, the decision whether or not to wear a cuff is a matter of personal choice. Most people feel that cuffs are more conservative/dressy, therefore would be out of place on a pair of dress slacks or more obviously, a pair of jeans. A sleek, European-style suit with a pair of beautiful Italian leather shoes would not be consistent with cuffs on the pant bottoms. The opposite would be true of a fine English or American business suit with a classic cap toe shoe. Here, a cuff would be elegant and perfectly in place. If the decision of cuffing is to be based on camouflaging, here is a simple guide. To elongate the leg, choose cuffless pants; to minimize long legs, choose to have a cuff added.

The width of the cuff is not a very serious issue. As long as it isn't so wide as to look like you were accompanying the Duke of Windsor through a walk in the muddy fields and trying to protect your trouser bottoms or the other extreme of a slim, little sliver which is hardly worth the effort, you can't err too much. If you're looking for a rule try this: use the width of the belt loops as a balance, stay within ¼-inch of this and you'll always be safe.

Pockets Bowing Out

We all have an age that we sort of think of ourselves as being. It may be 21, 25, 30, 35, or whatever. I truly feel that this is perfectly natural and harmless. Many men seem to want to do this with their pant size as well. This causes disaster.

If a few extra pounds have crept into a guy's waistline, which is where it seems to go on men, there is no way to wear your old pants the way they were meant to be worn. It produces what I refer to as the "ice cream cone effect," thin tapered bottom bulging to roundness above.

Before you reach this point there is a period of warning. If you watch for it, you may be able to take action before you get too far out of hand. When you look at yourself in the mirror, look at the front pant pockets especially closely. Regardless whether they are on seam, diagonal, or horizontal they should lie close, fairly flat to the material on the edge of the opening, touching.

If the pockets bow out, the pants are trying to compensate for slightly more than they were meant to hold. Don't fall for the trap of wearing too snug pants, expecting them to provide inspiration which will result in lost weight.

Lose the weight or have them let out. Or buy a pair of "fat pants" to wear until you can wear the smaller size.

Horizontal Creases Across Front

A certain amount of room is built into a man's trousers so that he can sit and bend and stoop comfortably. When that built-in reserve begins to be filled up with person, it exhibits a series of horizontal lines across the lap after sitting or bending for a prolonged period of time. If the pants are made of good natural fabric, these lines will fall out in time when properly hung.

Too Small Waist Size

Buying and wearing a size 34-waist pant when a tape measure reads 36 when wrapped around you does not make you look thinner. It actually contributes to that male malady—the spare tire. You will actually appear thinner if your pants fit, regardless of the numbers sewn into the waistband. This is because instead of squeezing any excess up above the waistband (I've never seen anyone squeeze it down) you simply cover it and your pants can ride in the proper position. This also allows the pant leg to fall properly.

The temptation to deceive seems universal. If we wore size 34 five years ago and can get into them today, then we must be in as good shape as we were then. The wearer is the only one who is ever fooled. The fact that the pants' waistband is worn 3½ inches lower than it used to be is conveniently overlooked. A glance downward to where the cuff used to gently break as it just touched the shoe's instep, is now a cascade of material bagged up like an elephant's ankles.

If time and gravity have taken their toll, then the only thing short of exercise and diet is to go up in size. Only your dry cleaner will know for sure.

What to Look for When Having Trousers Fitted

- Trousers should fit at the waist. Unlike jeans that fit *at* the hips, trousers need the hips to provide the support that keeps them in place. The most important variable to be aware of is the rise (the distance between the base of the crotch and the waistband). The rise can vary from one manufacturer to another, so do not compromise. You cannot be comfortable if the rise is incorrect for your body type.

- If you choose to wear suspenders (also called braces), allow an extra half-inch in the waist to accommodate the "hardware"—the buttons and pig-skin tabs. Belted or side-tab model trousers should be just snug enough to stay up. Insert one finger between you and the waistband to ensure comfort.

- Pockets and pleats do not bow open or pull apart when standing erect. Pleats do have a functional basis. They were created to combine a styling detail and added comfort. The hips widen when we are seated. The pleats allow the trouser fabric to do likewise.

- The trouser seat may be altered to fit looser or more snugly. But be careful: these alterations usually affect the crotch's fit somewhat.

- Pant bottoms "break" at the shoe tops. Avoid the two extremes of "high water pants" and "elephant ankles." High-waters mean the bottoms don't reach the shoes. Elephant ankles means folds of fabric that billow over the foot. The correct length is a bit more than just touching the shoe tops. A safe rule of thumb is: trousers must be long enough to cover your socks when you walk.

- Cuffs, should you choose to wear them, should be about one-and-a-half-inches wide. There is some debate as to whether cuffs are appropriate for a short man. I believe in the end it is a matter of personal choice. Cuffs do provide more weight and pull to anchor the pant bottoms and make them drape properly.

- Cuffed bottoms should be hemmed straight across. Uncuffed bottoms should be hemmed about one-half-inch longer in the back.

- It is always dangerous to let down a cuffless trouser leg due to the ironed-in hem. It's suggested that if you must lower a cuffless bottom, convert it into a cuff that will help camouflage the previous hem.

Costly thy habit as thy purse can buy,
But not express'd in fancy; rich not gaudy
For the apparel oft proclaims the man.

William Shakespeare
Hamlet

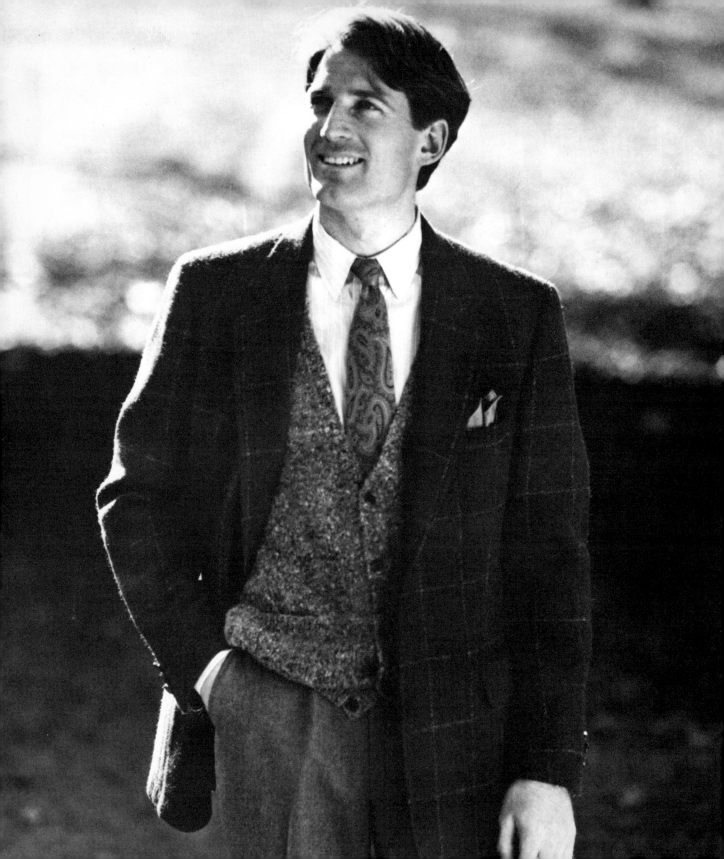

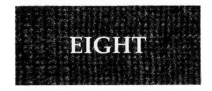

EIGHT

The Ties Have It

Tying the Best One On

Axiom: There's no such thing as a "well, it's okay" tie. Ties either work for you or they work against you—with a vengance!

It's also a fact that many men delegate the chore of picking their ties to three women in their lives: wives, lovers, and secretaries. Mothers and sisters also contribute their fair share to a man's tie rack. Now a number of men will shrug, "But women have an eye for these things. They're more 'sensitive' to color." There may be some truth to this. But the logic is debatable and to exercise it constantly is to rob yourself of the skills you need to master your *own* selection of this extremely important item of apparel. No pain, no gain; use it or lose it. It's up to you. You probably don't send the women in your life out to buy your automobile and you shouldn't be passing the buck when it comes to an item that is considered "you."

What follows, then, is a series of checkpoints that will help you make your choices, and a list of little "uglies" you're to avoid.

If you're one of the great number of men who are accustomed to leaving their apparel selections to the women in their lives, it may be a good idea to shop with them and learn what it is that gives them a special eye. Later, strike out on your own and try it yourself. You'll be surprised how really good you are at making selections that constitute perfect taste and—equally important—

picking the neckwear that subtly expresses what is special about the inner man.

Here are the insider's tips of the trade. Use them for your own winner's style:

Three or More Patterns in One Tie

Often, a misguided attempt to produce a necktie that will appeal to everyone ends up a designer's nightmare, a tie that should appeal to no one. Consider a tie with one-inch bars in a foulard pattern (evenly spaced, very small geometric print). After a short, solid space it changes into several coordinated colors of stripes, then on the same solid color background, a duck in flight bursts forth from the wearer's stomach.

Unless the wearer's name is "Daffy," he should simply retire his tacky "friend."

Many excellent books have been written on the rules for combining patterns when dressing. Some say to combine three solids: it's the safest way. Others tell how to work with two solids and one pattern; or one solid and two patterns. Some fashion magazines even show an interesting look when combining three patterns, though this is considered a little too fashionable for most business situations.

Tie Tying Troubles

There are three ways to botch it in this very visible area of dressing:

First is the tie's fabrication. If the tie has a lot of polyester in it, it has a heavier lining to keep its shape. Hence, a very out-of-proportion knot results.

Second, the Windsor knot (a large knot popularized by the late Duke of Windsor and, more recently, by Ronald Reagan), is very formal, symmetrical, and extremely stylish when worn with a spread collar. It should not be worn with button-down collars or a collar bar, pin or tab collar.

Third, if the ends of your tie are nearly even before you begin the knot, odds are that when you finish the knot it will not be the proper length. If you are of average height, the wide end of your tie should be approximately 9½–10½ inches longer when first draped around your neck before you begin to tie it.

---

*A well tied tie
is the first
serious step in life.*

Oscar Wilde

Tie Too Short

Most ties are made to measure 56½ inches when laid out end-to-end. If you happen to be the exact size the tie manufacturer had in mind, your tie would end just at the top of your belt buckle or ever so slightly below the top. If, however, your tie falls neatly down from your collar to your chest only to leap out at right angles from your body when it reaches your stomach, you need to do some adjusting.

A "pot belly" is most often the reason for a significant gap between the tie and belt line. Many of us are trying desperately to continue wearing the size 34-inch pants of yesteryear. Not only would losing the extra girth make the loved one in your life incredibly happy, it will likely solve the too-short tie problem for you.

Wearing pants that fit just below the navel (where they belong) helps, too. If you absolutely refuse to do either, then observe how much of a gap you have from the tip of the wide end of your tie to the top of your belt. Increase the length of the tie's wider end before tying by this amount. Assuming the discrepancy isn't great, this should do it.

When tied, the narrow end should still fit through the loop on the back of your tie to help keep it in place. If not, a qualified tailor can move the loop for you.

If your tie is *still* too short, you should investigate the big and tall men's shops for ties specially designed for the bigger guy.

Hula Dancers Belong in Hawaii, Not in Your Tie

A man's necktie is supposed to say something about who he is or who he would like to be. Some men buy ties with designer labels on the outside. This message may say to others that you've given up and are content to let that glaring label say, "I've got good taste, just like Pierre Cardin . . ."

In a business setting a tie should never advertise, should not be the backdrop for gaudy patterns and colors. Having said this, we now present the eight most common patterns for neckties, with enough variety to please the most eclectic or discriminating of men. How they all work with shirts and suits will be discussed later on. For now, here's the basic neckwear menu:

Solid

A single color in silk, wool, cotton, or a blend of fibers. A "must have" for all men.

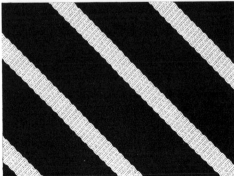

Striped

Sometimes called a rep stripe, regimental, or school tie. In England it is poor form to wear the stripes of a regiment in which you did not serve.

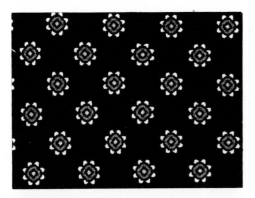

Foulard

Made up of a series of small, regularly spaced designs such as circles, ovals, diamonds, or a combination of shapes on a solid background.

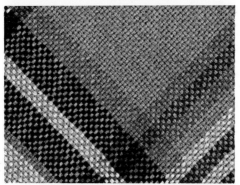

Plaid

Usually of wool for winter wear or cotton for summer, they are generally considered casual.

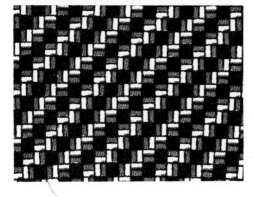

Geometric

This can be everything from an enlarged diamond pattern to a crisscross or vertically striped pattern.

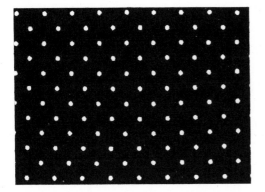

Dots

Ranging downward in size from approximately the diameter of a dime to mini- and micro-dots.

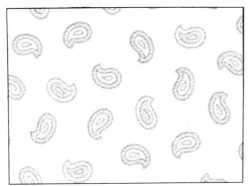

Paisley

These can go from very sporty if the colors are bright, to very elegant if the colors are subdued. Because of the combination of colors, this pattern can go with a variety of items in clothing.

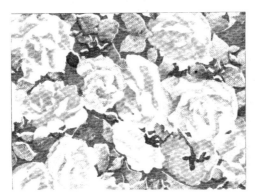

Floral

This pattern is showing up on businessmen in more "fashion forward" cities such as New York and Los Angeles. Be careful, it hasn't yet become part of the basic business "uniform."

Tie Too Wide or Too Narrow

Pierre Cardin was quoted as saying, "In men's fashion, the look changes every five years. But on the streets, it changes every ten years." Don't take this designer's very astute observation and distort it to mean that you can put a tie in the back of your closet, pull it out a decade later, wear it, and assume no one will know it's ten years old. They *will* know it's old; don't do it!

Tie widths correspond very closely to the width of a man's suit or sport coat lapels. To tell if a tie is appropriate with a particular jacket, hold the wide end of your tie up against the widest part of the jacket's lapel. The tie should not be wider than the lapel. It can be a bit narrower, but not too much.

If you have a prized possession that you don't want to part with, take advantage of the cost-effective services of a qualified tailor who will recut your old pal to today's standards of between 2¾ inches–3½ inches. If you are unable to find someone in your area, two companies that can help are:

Tiecrafters, Inc.   Lords Tiecrafter Division
116 E. 27th Street   Mark Morris & Co., Inc.
New York, New York 10016   1825T Chicago
                                         Minneapolis, MN 55404

Horizontal Crease Across Tie

You may wonder why some men's neckties have a line, a crease actually, about thre-fourths of the way down their length. Well, at the end of a particularly grueling day hunched over my desk working on a speech I was to deliver, I checked myself out in the mirror before leaving. By trapping my tie between stomach and desk and applying pressure for several hours, voilá—a big crease. Though in the scheme of things, this isn't that serious a problem because your buttoned jacket or vest will cover it, you should try to prevent it from becoming a permanent part of your "look." If it is a problem for you, I would not recommend trying to press the crease out at home. Do try a little steam, but be careful that you don't overdo it. Too much can cause the lining to sag which equals a ruined tie.

Unfortunately, finding a competent tie-cleaning professional is no easy task prompting one men's clothing authority to comment that sending a tie to many cleaners is the same as throwing it in the trash and then paying up to four dollars for your trouble.

Cotton/Wool Knit Tie with a Business Suit

Consistency of fabrics is a very subtle art to be learned when combining articles of clothing. Generally you cannot assume that two items belong together because they are made of the same material. It may depend on the formality of the fabrics. A wool or wool-blend suit usually calls for a silk-blend tie. A Harris Tweed sport coat would be terribly out of place with a silk shantung tie.

Neckties are at their best when made out of silk or a high quality blend. When they are made out of wool, cotton, or linen, they become more casual and should therefore be worn with a blazer or sport coat.

Tie Longer than Belt Line

Because tie lengths vary only slightly, there are only a few variables to note: The circumference of your neck ("average" is considered to be 15½ inches); the type of knot that you are tying (four-in-hand, half-Windsor, or full Windsor) and the ratio of narrow end to wide before you begin to form the knot.

As your neck size is unlikely to change significantly, before you tie your tie, allow a bit more wide-to-narrow ratio when you drape it around your neck.

If you decide to try a different knot than the one you're used to, be prepared to experiment with the location of the thin end of your tie. Usually, a four-in-hand knot will leave the tip of your thin end at your fourth button. Once you establish this relationship it shouldn't change.

The full Windsor, because of its double wrap, uses more fabric than the half-Windsor, which in turn takes more material than the four-in-hand.

Narrow End Longer than Wide End

There is no excuse for this to happen. It takes about 10 seconds to tie a necktie, so if you end up with the thin end peeking out, undo it by reversing the steps used to tie it, pull the wide end a bit farther down (approximately half the amount of the thin end that was showing), and start again.

Worst case, if you absolutely can't get it right, at least do this: tuck the thin end into your shirt. Spare the world from this terrible dressing faux pas. One last word, we are not talking degrees of bad here. No amount, not even one inch, should show. Not for a man with winner's style.

Tie Tacks

A tie tack is just what the name implies. It has a pointed end that you push through the center of both ends of your necktie. Though the everyday variety has a flat or rounded head, most tie tacks are fancier. Many are embellished with monograms, diamonds, or pearls. In order to accomplish its mission—namely to hold the tie in place—the pointed end has to be pushed into something and, fortunately, the inventors did not choose your chest. Instead, it fits into a small metal clip that is connected by a fine chain to a bar that fits into your button hole.

Men seem to either wear tie tacks frequently—and if that's their personal statement, that's okay—or they almost never wear one. Owning a tie tack though, can be something of a self-fulfilling prophecy. Once you have decided to wear it, you must *always* wear it as it puts a hole in the center of your tie. It does limit your dressing options, which is not usually an advantage, especially with a fine silk tie that costs $30 to $50. Poking a hole in its most visible part is a shame!

Bow Ties: Can They be Worn for Business?

The answer is a qualified yes. You will find very successful men who prefer the bow tie over the more conventional cravat in just about every profession. But because it's a very visible form of expression, be sure that it is in keeping with the image you wish to convey. If you are in a somewhat creative field, the bow tie will convey an air of uniqueness. An academic will send out the message "I am an independent thinker." For much more practical reasons, doctors who choose to wear a bow tie claim it doesn't get in their way when examining a patient. Just be aware of the circumstances and act accordingly.

Tying a Bow Tie

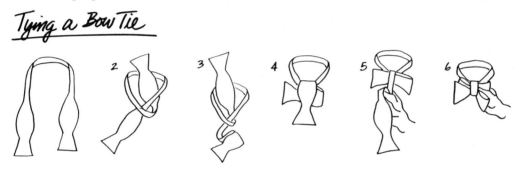

"*A woman should not play too large a role
in the clothes that a man wears.
Men who have
learned how to mix patterns have mastered
something very important.
A tie is one of the
best forms of self-expression a man has, so
why should his wife pick it?*"

Bill Blass
New York Times Magazine
September 16, 1984

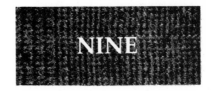

NINE

An Introduction to Color

In 1981, Acropolis Books published the best-selling *Color Me Beautiful** by Carole Jackson, giving millions the opportunity to logically identify colors that make them look their best. This system is called the "Seasonal Color Theory," and is based on the premise that each of us has a certain skin tone, hair, and eye color that can be identified as being a part of one of four groups. These groups are named after the seasons. You are either a *Winter, Summer, Autumn,* or *Spring.*

Your "season" has nothing to do with when you were born or any astrological signs—there's no mystery to it at all! Your "season" never changes, not as you grow older or when you have a tan. Take a look at the following groups and find where you fit.

- **Winters** have dark coloring or strong contrast between the color of their skin, eyes, and hair. They usually have dark brown or black hair. (cool undertones)
- **Summers** are fair, and have less contrast between the color of their skin, eyes, and hair. They have visible pink in their complexions, and light brown to sandy blonde hair. (cool undertones)
- **Autumns** have dark coloring with golden skin undertones, and usually have red hair or at least red highlights in their hair. (warm undertones)
- **Springs,** lighter versions of Autumns, are more delicate and fair. Their skin is golden or ivory and they tend to have light red to golden blonde hair. (warm undertones)

*An updated edition is now available from your bookseller at $14.95, or directly from Acropolis Books Ltd., 2400 17th St., NW, Washington, DC 20009. Add $2.00 for shipping. Call TOLL-FREE 800-621-5199 24 hours/7 days.

What are warm colors and cool colors?

Being able to identify colors as warm or cool is important in choosing clothes and accessories for a coordinated wardrobe.

- *Warm colors* have more yellow in them. For instance, a certain green that is more yellow than other choices is a warmer green.
- *Cool colors* have less yellow in them. For instance, a certain green that is less yellow than other choices is a cooler green.

Cool Greens	**Warm Greens**

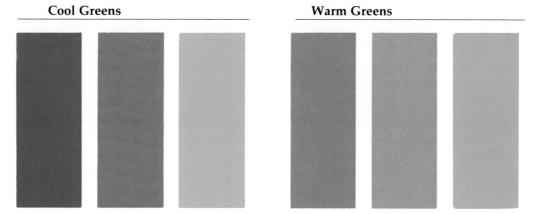

Note how the cool greens look less yellow and the warm greens look more yellow. This is the same relationship you will notice among various types of all colors.

Winter and Summers should always choose cool colors.

Autumns and Springs should always choose warm colors.

Look at the Color Planners on the following pages. Compare the Winter and Summer Color Planners (*cool*) to the Autumn and Spring Color Planners (*warm*).

Which Seasonal Grouping do you fall into?

On each of the following Color Planner pages, look for the Eye Color and Hair Color lists. Decide which of the four is the best description of you. Then study your colors.

Winter

Winter's clothes have a strength and simplicity about them. A Winter man is dashing in a dark navy suit, a bright white broadcloth shirt, and a brilliant red silk tie.

"Dark," "Bright," "Clear," and "Strong Contrast" are characteristics that describe a Winter's color choices.

Eye Colors

dark brown
almost black
gray-blue
violet
turquoise
green

Hair Colors

black
dark brown
deep brown mixed
with red
silvery gray
very white

Winter People

George Hamilton
Pierce Brosnan
Omar Sharif
Eddie Murphy
Gene Shalit

COLOR PLANNER

Dark: Suits, Sports Jackets and Slacks

Light: Shirts (Solid and Striped)

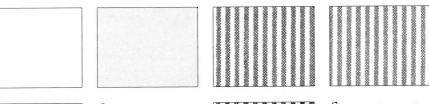

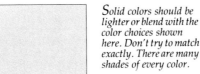

Solid colors should be lighter or blend with the color choices shown here. Don't try to match exactly. There are many shades of every color.

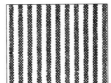

Stripes can be any color in your Planner. Many colors that are too dark to be worn as a solid shirt look fine as a stripe against a light background.

Bright: Ties, Accents and Sportswear

Summer

Summers are lighter than Winters. They have less contrast between skin, hair, and eyes. Summer colors give a look of cool, calm and control. A slightly grayed navy suit with white or pastel oxfordcloth shirt is best for Summers. For the tie, red is fine, but not a vibrant shade. Go for a more subdued red, one that doesn't shout across the room.

Eye Colors

blue
gray-blue
green
light aqua
hazel

Hair Colors

sandy blonde
light brown
dark brown
silvery gray

Summer People

Paul Newman
Don Johnson
John Ritter
Johnny Carson
Philip Michael Thomas

COLOR PLANNER

Dark: Suits, Sports Jackets and Slacks

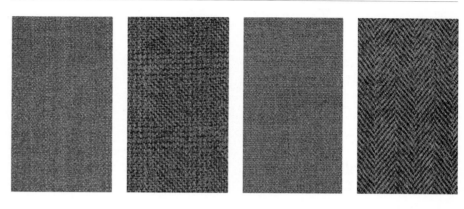

Light: Shirts (Solid and Striped)

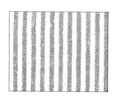
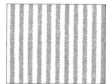

Solid colors should be lighter or blend with the color choices shown here. Don't try to match exactly. There are many shades of every color.

Stripes can be any color in your Planner. Many colors that are too dark to be worn as a solid shirt look fine as a stripe against a light background.

Bright: Ties, Accents and Sportswear

Autumn

COLOR PLANNER

Autumn's best colors are browns, rusts, greens. His best blue suit is a warm, almost teal-toned blue. Avoid bright shirts; they will drain color from the face. Autumns look best in light blues, or oyster white shirts with stripes in accent colors. Ties should incorporate these accent colors and blend with the outfit, avoiding strong contrasts.

Dark: Suits, Sports Jackets and Slacks

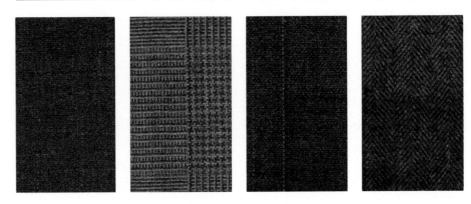

Eye Colors

brown
green
amber
turquoise
hazel

Light: Shirts (Solid and Striped)

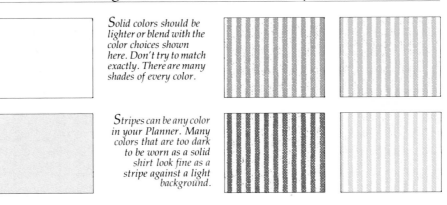

Solid colors should be lighter or blend with the color choices shown here. Don't try to match exactly. There are many shades of every color.

Stripes can be any color in your Planner. Many colors that are too dark to be worn as a solid shirt look fine as a stripe against a light background.

Hair Colors

red
coppery
golden blonde
golden brown
charcoal black
golden gray

Autumn People

Robert Redford
David Hartman
George Siegal
Danny Kaye
Red Buttons
Red Skelton

Bright: Ties, Accents and Sportswear

Spring

Spring men look best in clear, bright colors. This season is the toughest to dress in "typical" business attire because the usual business look, serious colors, are not his best ones. A Spring's best business color is a blue that virtually "jumps" with life. (Compare the blue in the American flag to a dark navy blue.) Springs should wear ivory, or off-white shirts. Springs are lucky in the tie department. They may choose from dozens of colorful combinations.

Eye Colors

bright blue
aqua
bright green
light brown
blue-gray

Hair Colors

blonde
golden brown
golden blonde
auburn
gold-gray

Spring People

Dick Cavett
Ron Howard
Jimmy Carter
David Letterman
Ed Begley, Jr.

COLOR PLANNER

Dark: Suits, Sports Jackets and Slacks

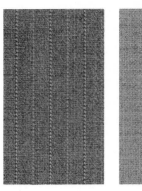 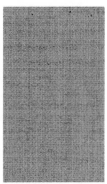 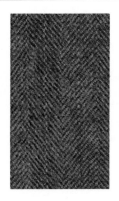 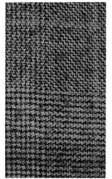

Light: Shirts (Solid and Striped)

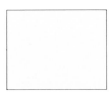

Solid colors should be lighter or blend with the color choices shown here. Don't try to match exactly. There are many shades of every color.

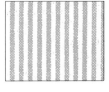 

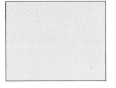

Stripes can be any color in your Planner. Many colors that are too dark to be worn as a solid shirt look fine as a stripe against a light background.

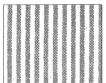 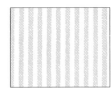

Bright: Ties, Accents and Sportswear

Q: I'm choosing a tie. Which one should I get?

A: Each season has its own correct answer. Your choice is determined by whether you are a Winter, Summer, Autumn, or Spring.

1. Winter   2. Summer   3. Autumn   4. Spring

1—Winter's best reds are deep, blue-reds.   2—Summer's best reds are lighter and pinker.   3—Autumn's best reds are more yellow and deep.   4—Spring's best reds are lighter, more orange.

Q: I'm choosing a sweatshirt. Which should I get?

A: 1—Winter's best blues are dark.   2.—Summer's best blues are lighter.   3—Autumn's best blues are teal.   4—Spring's best blues are aqua.

1. Winter   2. Summer   3. Autumn   4. Spring

Q: I'm choosing a sweater. Which is right for me?

A: 1—Winter's best yellow is bright and clear.   2—Summer's best yellows are soft.   3—Autumn's best yellows are golden and deep.   4—Spring's best yellows are bright and golden.

1. Winter   2. Summer   3. Autumn   4. Spring

Q: I'm choosing a new pair of khakis. Which khaki is right for me?

A: Winters and Summers should choose a non-yellow khaki. Autumns and Springs should choose a yellow, golden khaki.

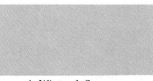 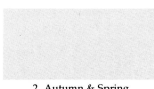

1. Winter & Summer   2. Autumn & Spring

Q: Do colors really make that much of a difference?

A: Choosing colors correctly for your wardrobe can make a big difference. Some benefits are:

- Clearer understanding of what is best for you
- Increased confidence in your product selection
- Prevents mistakes when shopping, and saves you money
- Greater ease in explaining your needs and desires to salespeople
- Enhances appearance—you will look better
- Establishes a solid foundation for your wardrobe, and expands your possible combinations
- Makes dressing foolproof, because all items coordinate
- Saves time while getting dressed

Q: Do I have to find an exact match?

A: No. Look for a good blend, remembering—"Is it the right warm or cool choice for me?"

Q: How do I coordinate my shoes with my clothing colors?

A: Black, brown, or burgundy (cordovan) will work in virtually every business situation. For fun clothes, try a color that matches or blends with your sport slacks.

Q: What about socks?

A: For business, your socks should almost always match or be darker than your slacks. Don't limit yourself to black. Try medium or dark gray, navy, or brown if those are the suit colors you wear most often. For casual wear, match either your slacks or shirt.

Q: What if some of the colors in my tie are not in my Color Planner?

A: The base color of your tie is the main consideration. If that works with your suit and shirt, then you will look great. Small amounts of other colors add interest and variety to your winning look.

Q: Isn't this color system limiting?

A: Actually, it encourages you to try many colors. The colors presented in your Color Planner are just the beginning. A qualified color consultant can teach you to incorporate hundreds of shades into your wardrobe.

Q: Some of the colors in my Color Planner seem too dark for business shirts. What should I look for?

A: For solid shirts, find shades that are lighter or blend with your recommended colors. Don't try to reproduce them exactly! For striped shirts, find your white as a background and look for stripes in your best colors.

Q: I've heard a lot about skin tone. What does it mean?

A: Everyone has either a blue or a golden skin tone. If your underlying color is blue-based, you look best in what are called cool colors (blue or pink-based). If your skin color is golden, you need the warm or yellow/gold-based colors to bring out your best.

Q: Should I wear gold or silver jewelry?

A: Winters and Summers should wear silver. Autumns and Springs are best in gold. Since most men wear so little jewelry—a wedding ring and a watch—just continue to wear your old favorites.

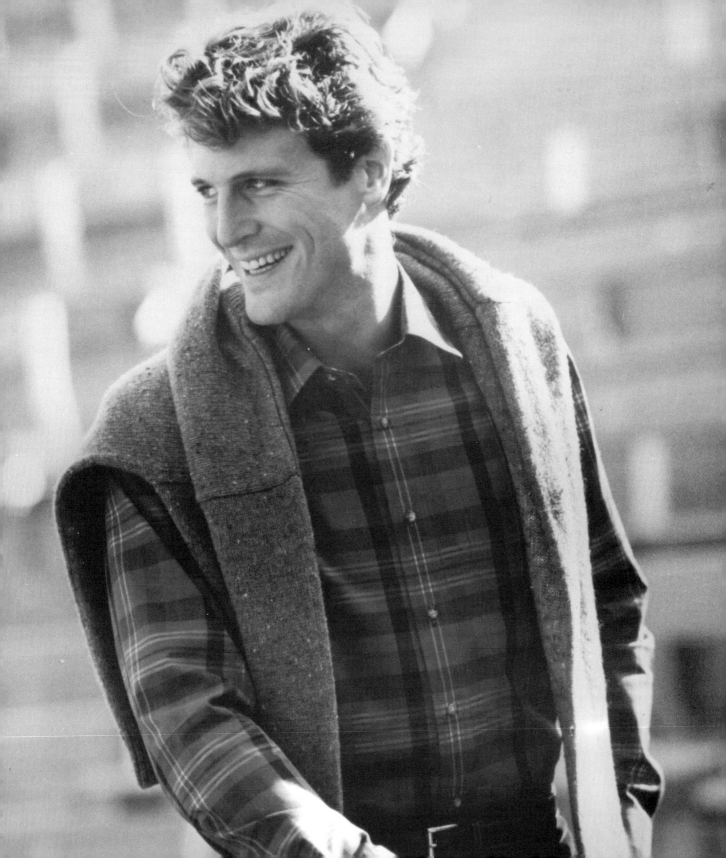

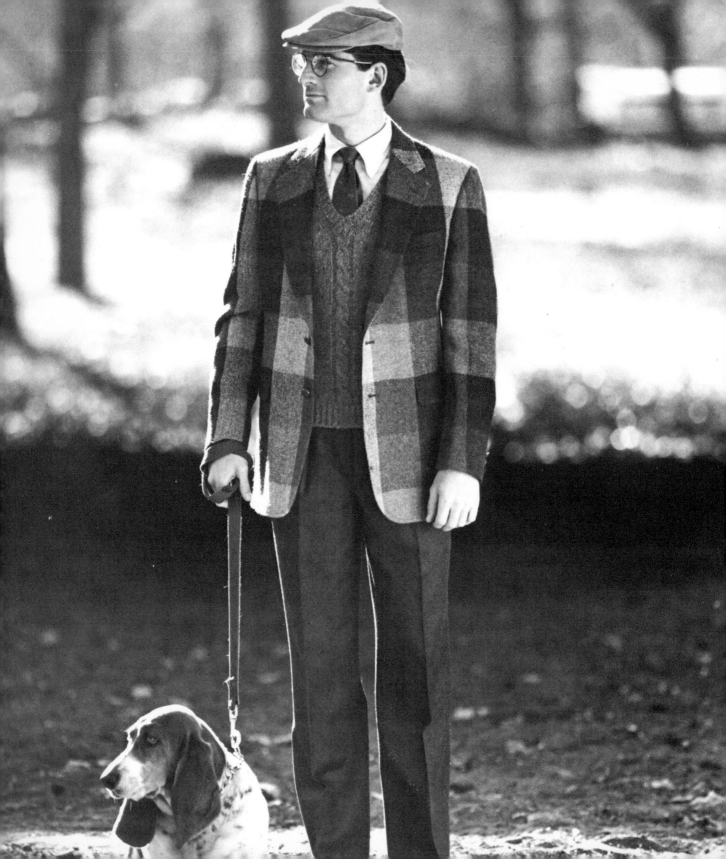

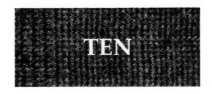

TEN

Down to the Toes: Shoes and Socks

If the Shoe Fits . . .

It is said that if you want to know if a man is truly well-dressed, "look down."

Below the perfect break of a man's perfectly made trouser cuffs are his shoes, and if they're out of sync with the rest of him, his winner's look will end abruptly. The rules tend to be painfully hard and fast: your shoes must be right. Quality must be excellent. Fashion must be minimal. Style must be quietly and elegantly right for the occasion. Period!

Of course, there's a good deal of latitude outside the office—everything from hi-tech sports shoes to the patent leather pumps of a royal coronation. Still, shoes simply must fit the moment.

It is a false economy at best—foolhardy at worst—to scrimp on your footwear. When it comes to spending a few extra dollars for the best quality, don't hesitate. You won't invest in flaky penny stocks if you're after a high-quality portfolio, and shoes are one of the highest values in any winner's sartorial collection. You won't regret it.

How to Buy Shoes

Men's shoes are one of the best values around today, dollar for dollar. With proper care they will last for years. Periodic replacement of soles and heels, along with regular polishing with both a cream and a wax polish, and finally, regular rest periods with a pair of good shoe trees in place will allow you to amortize the original price over many years. All the care in the world will not help if you do not make certain your shoes fit you in the first place. Here are eight tips to help you get a perfect fit.

- Shop after you have been out and about a bit, since feet do swell. This way you will get the most realistic measurement.
- Shop only at a store that uses a Brannock foot measuring device for determining your exact foot size.
- Almost everyone has one foot larger than the other, usually it is the right foot; fit the shoes to the larger right foot. Do not rely solely on the size you have always worn. Different makers can vary significantly from each other, even though the numeric size is the same. Buy them by how they feel on your feet.
- Allow a half-inch between the tips of your toes and your shoes. If the toes of the shoes are pointed, be certain there is enough room for your toes to move comfortably. Shoes should never be tight over the instep or ball of the foot.
- When considering an oxford-style shoe, you should not be able to tie the laces so tightly that the two edges of the shoe meet. If you can, a narrower size is probably better for you.
- Buy leather shoes. Though more expensive, because it is porous, leather is the best for the health and comfort of your feet. In leather shoes the foot can breathe, discouraging the build-up of bacteria.
- Shoes should fit from the moment you try them on. Do not accept the salesperson's, "Once you break them in they will be fine." The man-made materials used today do not stretch significantly, but leather adapts to your foot shape quite well.
- When shopping, wear the same type of sock you will use with the dress or sport shoes. Too heavy or too thin socks will distort the fit.

Quality Upkeep

A professional shoe shine is worth much more than what you pay for it. Consider two points:

1. If you're after a winner's style and you've invested good money in your shoes, it's really unbecoming to be shy about a professional shine.

2. If your inner voice tells you it's demeaning for the bootblack to be performing such a service, ask your inner voice why the bootblack is doing it in the first place. The answer is that it's profitable and—if you want the real truth—it's an old and honored profession.

If you're a do-it-yourselfer, here's a step-by-step guide to getting the kind of shine your drill instructor would approve of:

Polishing Shoes

- Cream polish such as Meltonian Cream feeds fine leather and keeps it supple. Wax polish like Kiwi Wax Polish which brings up a shine and is somewhat water resistant, will also do a good job. Both polishes come in a wide range of colors.

- Before polishing be sure to remove all dust and surface dirt. You'll need a cloth to use with cream polish, and for wax-type polish, a small circular brush for application and a separate larger one for the actual polishing will do the job.

- When polishing you may prefer to leave your shoe trees inside the shoes, providing a smoother and more stable surface to work with.

The following method is used by a number of military institutions as well as shoe shine professionals:

- Apply polish to one shoe with an applicator. Allow it to soak in while you apply a coat of polish to the other shoe.

- Wrap the corner of a clean cloth around your first and second fingers. Twist the rest of the cloth into a spiral and tighten the section around your fingers. Hold onto the spiral in the palm of your hand.

- Dab the cloth lightly along the surface of the polish.

- Rub the polish into the toe in a circular motion. As the surface dries out and the cloth begins to drag, spit lightly on the shoe. (If you've been eating or drinking sweets or dairy products this can become messy. Instead, use a spray mister or put a few drops of water in the lid of your polish container and dip the applicator in that.)
- Continue to add polish, a little at a time, and cover the entire shoe.
- Very lightly buff the shoe with the polishing brush (most of the best are made out of horse hair). This will bring out the shine, so don't press too firmly.
- Finally, using a soft, clean cloth, rub briskly back and forth to bring out a high luster.

Footwear Etiquette

The following pages will provide you with the dos and don'ts you'll need to make you a "shoe-in" for the winner's style.

Unpolished Shoes

Anyone who walks around with shoes that look as though they were buffed-up using a brick and a Hershey bar is telling the world they just don't care. Not a pretty picture. Not caring bespeaks an attitude that has no place in the business or professional community. So our message is: keep a shine.

Gunboat-Style Shoes

A special note to recently separated military types: The Armed Forces issue a good quality, long-wearing shoe to its personnel and it is easy to think of it as an acceptable piece of civilian-wear after separation. Not true. Don't fall into this trap. A proper pair of business shoes should have a sole with a thickness of ⅝-inch or less. Look at the stitches on the top of the sole. The most expensive, as well as most familiar, method of attaching the sole to the uppers is referred to as the Goodyear welt. It is a grooved effect that runs around the shoe. Usually, inexpensive or sporty shoes won't use this method. Of course, few people will carefully examine your shoe's soles, but you'll know.

Check the inner lining, which should also be leather, and the uppers, which should also be leather. Top-quality cowhide and calfskin are good choices, as is cordovan. Avoid most man-made fabrics and anything that looks as though small planes could take off from them.

Dress Shoes and Casual Attire

Avoid making mistakes in this area by learning what goes with what. Shoes that are at home with a business suit should not be worn with jeans, casual pants such as linen blends or ducks, and most positively not with Bermuda shorts.

Slip-on shoes present a minefield full of potential problems when worn with a suit. There is a tassled loafer seen in the business community on stockbrokers, retailers, and people in the clothing industry. It is considered an acceptable look for these and other non-conservative occupations, yet only a top-quality cowhide or cordovan model will do. The economy models just don't cut it. Penny loafers are best not worn with suits. Youngsters can pull this off, but it can be considered improper. Shoes like penny loafers, Topsiders,™ and most slip-ons belong with slacks and open-collared sport shirt or even a sport coat and tie. Athletic shoes have a clear cut place. If you are ever tempted to wear your Nikes with your suit, the way that many young female professionals have, don't do it.

Boots with a Suit

There is such a thing as a dress boot but few men know about them and fewer still own and wear them. We will not discuss them here. Chukkas, desert boots, and a line that is synonymous with quality—Frye—do not have a place in a business setting, unless you are mapping out the lease area of your next oil and gas venture in the Oklahoma Panhandle.

Alligator Nipping at Your Heels

A recent informal poll revealed that one of the major differences between men and women and how they rank important items of apparel, is in shoes and their maintenance. Some women complain that they have no shoes to wear while surveying 75 pairs sitting nearly untouched in the original boxes. A pair for every conceivable occasion except, of course, the one they need to be shod for at the moment.

Conversely, a man will own a total of three pair of shoes and try to make them work with everything. The problem arises as his business pair begins to wear down. He knows that having them repaired will leave him without them for about a week. Because he has an important meeting scheduled for the middle of the week, he puts it off until the following weekend. This goes on and on until he comes upon a "While-U-Wait" repair shop, usually by chance. Don't let this happen to you. If you can put your shoe on a flat surface with the eraser end of a pencil against the heel and the eraser fits under, they are in need of repair. Replace the heels once in a while; it's a very cost-effective way to make them last.

"Hard work alone isn't enough. Men are watching people being promoted above them, and they wonder why they're not moving too. One reason is that they just don't look as promotable."

Susan Bixler
Author, *The Professional Image* (Putnam)
Success Magazine

Skin Showing When Seated

Whose fault is it that, despite well-meaning advice, men are still exposing their hairy/semi-hairy calves to the world? More than anything else, it's due to modern science. Before the perfection of man-made elasticized socks, silk, cotton, or wool socks really had no way to stay up on a man's leg. Garters were used for this purpose. The arrival of socks with an elastic band around the top was a God-send. Or was it? For comfort they were made shorter, as the synthetic band didn't "breathe." Then came all-synthetics, which had elastic mixed through the whole sock. The length stayed fairly short—not over the calf—again for comfort. These are fine socks, but the problem is that you simply can't "kill" them. Wash them repeatedly, bake them in a dryer, they just never seem in need of replacement. But replace them you should! If you can't remember when you bought them, seriously consider replacing them with a new pair of natural fiber socks. These contain only a small amount of elastic to keep them in place above the calf, and you will be amazed at how much better they feel and look.

Black Socks with Everything

When white socks fell out of favor in men's fashions, black socks took over. Men everywhere wore and continue to wear their black socks with everything. With a dark colored pair of pants as part of a business or dress look, they're no problem. But gentlemen, buy some different socks to wear with corduroys, bermuda shorts, and all of your favorite colored sport clothes. Jeans and black socks don't mix!

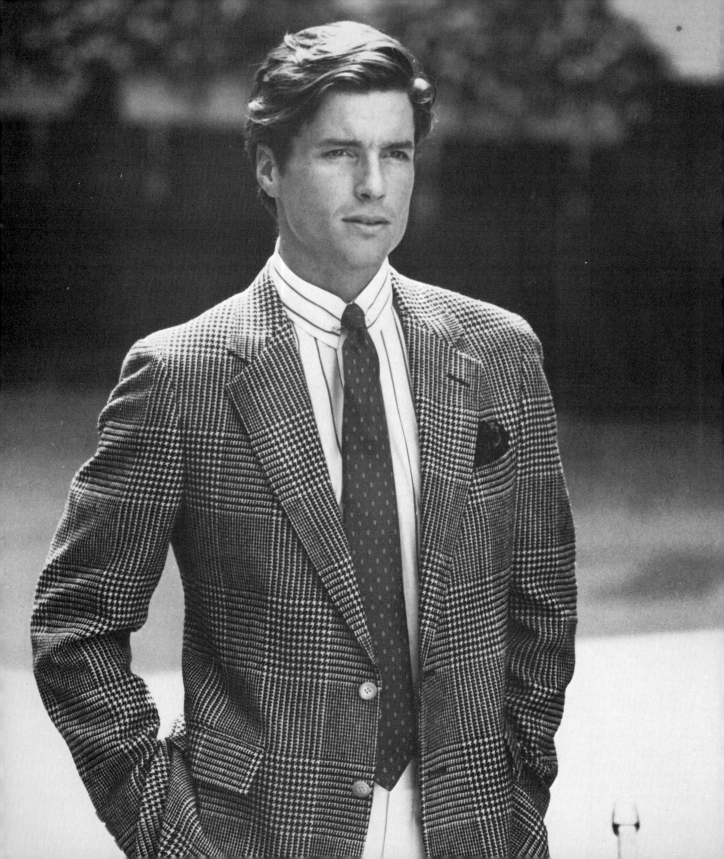

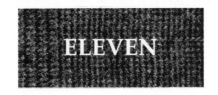

ELEVEN

Accessory Etiquette

All the "Little" Things Sure Add Up

Accessories—those casual items from pens to belts—can be the trickiest pieces of any man's wardrobe. They can ambush you, taking a big bite out of your style, so don't let it happen. You've invested a lot of time and money in your look. To allow all your good work and imagination to be ruined by a leaky ballpoint pen borders on the unforgivable, especially since such disasters are so avoidable.

The focus of this chapter is just that: *avoidance*, a crash course in sartorial damage control. And giving your accessories the respect they deserve will help you to keep your winner's style in top form. Let's begin in the good old pocketbook.

Fat Wallets

Turning your wallet into a micro-version of a woman's purse doesn't work. Decide what items are necessary each and every week and keep them handy. The others can be stored, ready to be called up when needed.

Men don't notice the fat-wallet syndrome on other men as often as women do. We men may not want to hear that where we carry our wallets (in our rear pant pocket) is an area closely scrutinized by many members of the opposite sex! This has less to do with matters sexual than it does physical fitness. When a woman sees a huge bulge where there should be a firm, tight package, it offends her sense of proportion. We are not born with, nor do we inherit, a wallet the size of a Big Mac; and yet, you will see them nearly everywhere you look. A recent check with a "good and true friend" (to borrow a phrase from my dear friend Sandy Hartman), revealed the following contents in his "ultra thin" wallet: an American Express company card, a magnetic card to open the garage door, a video club membership card, and the following credit cards—Choice, Bloomie's, MasterCard and Visa Silver, Shell Oil Co., Diners Club, Citibank Preferred, U.S. Air Club card. Also an electric banking card, a hospital insurance card, driver's license, health club membership, AAA membership card, 27 credit card receipts, and 3 pieces of paper with notes on them. All we can say is: WRONG! Pare it down to the minimum for the maximum look. Wallets aren't born fat; put yours on a diet!

Folding Your Pocket Square

Even though we won't make many friends in the coordinated tie and pocket hanky business, your tie and pocket square (which is how people in the business refer to the silk handkerchief worn in the breast pocket) should coordinate but not duplicate. If you choose to wear a pocket square, and I think it shows a definite dressing flair, then try to pull out one color, and repeat that in the square that you choose.

How you wear the silk pocket square is nearly as important as how it blends. There are many ways to fold a pocket square.

Since pocket squares can add so much to your total look, it's important to know how to wear them properly.

Here are the basic folds and how to do them:

- **The Puff.** Hold the square by its center, grasp the material with your other hand about half way down. Now, insert the points, which should be hanging straight down, into the pocket. Spread the fabric so it fills the pocket opening and only a "puff" of fabric shows.
- **The Flop.** Hold the fabric by its center, using the thumb and forefinger of your other hand circle the square as it hangs straight down. Slide your circling finger and thumb down a bit more than half way. Insert the square's center into the pocket allowing the points to fall freely or "flop" over.

- **The Plop.** Begin with the square completely open. Fold in half, and then in half again in order to form a smaller square. Pick up this smaller square by its center. With your other hand gently roll all of the loose points together. Once you've done that you should be holding a roughly cone-shaped piece of silk. Push the points into your jacket pocket and arrange the pointed top so that a dimple shows in the center.

- **Four-Point.** Start by folding the open square into an imperfect triangle. Next, fold up one of the lower corners so its point is separated by a few inches from the existing two points. By folding the other corner in the same way you'll have four points. Fold the base up and insert the pocket square into the pocket. Arrange the points to show all four clearly.

- **Three-Point.** Fold the square into a perfect triangle. Match the points carefully. Have the flat side toward you, the top of the triangle facing away. Move the lower left corner to the right of the top by a couple of inches. Next, move the right-hand corner to the left of the top. Adjust points so that they are even in height and spacing. Fold the bottom up about half way and push into your pocket.

- **TV Fold.** This is the simplest of all. Almost always done with a solid color handkerchief, it was very popular during the 1950s although it originated in the forties. When your handkerchief is folded to ⅛ its full size, just slip the side with the most edges into your pocket leaving about one-half to one inch showing above your pocket line. Be sure it's razor straight.

- **The Peaks.** Begin with the pocket square completely open. Fold over diagonally to form a perfect triangle with the flat side to your right. Fold edge C up just to the right of edge B and slightly higher. Now move edge A slightly higher and to the right of the two peaks at edge B. You should have a new triangle with the only difference three peaks at edge B. Fold point A over to become parallel with the flat side of the triangle. Next fold edge C up toward but just short of the peaks. Carefully slide the folded square into place. Adjust if necessary.

- **Arthur's Court.** Follow the instructions for folding a four-point pocket square given earlier. Once the points are formed, put one hand on the points and the other hand on the base. Now very carefully fold these two ends under the body of the square. The folds in the fabric should run parallel with the top of the breast pocket when inserted.

Pocketful of Pens

Whether or not the twelve pens are sheathed in a plastic case to protect the shirt from ink spots is really only a minor issue. There just isn't any reason to carry all of this artillery around. The average pen is more than capable of writing 10,000 words before giving up the ghost; very few people put even a fraction of that down on paper during any given day. Since volume is not a valid reason, that leads us to variety. Being able to make notations in living color or a range of lead thicknesses when away from one's desk doesn't seem very vital. If you need a writing instrument frequently, for signatures, brief notations, or some other reason, limit yourself to one pen and, if it is a matched set, one pencil. These should be of first-rate quality. After all, if you are using them so frequently, they should say something about you. Disposable pens do not convey a very positive impression.

For those of you who only remove your jackets while at your desks, try keeping your pen inside a coat pocket. Many manufacturers sew in a pen pocket on the left side of the lining, specifically for this purpose.

Captain Kangaroo Syndrome

From childhood right on through their golden years, men exhibit a nearly perverse love of pockets. Even a sophisticated sport coat can have as many as seven of them. For some, pockets are temporary storage areas; for others, they become treasure troves, yielding all sorts of wonderful things ranging from a forgotten $20.00 bill to the ticket stubs from last year's formal charity ball.

Whatever can logically be carried in a briefcase should be: extra pens, breath mints, calculator, etc. Keep the items on your person to the barest of minimums.

Most suits come with the outside pockets sewn shut. The simple reason is that the line of coats is cleaner without sagging or bulging pockets. If you need a little help to overcome the habit of loading things into your pockets, why not try leaving them sewn shut? Oxford, world famous clothing manufacturers, construct their pockets to bellow inward to help camouflage the Captain Kangaroo syndrome.

No "Gorilla-Proof" Briefcases Need Apply

No other accessory that a man can wear or carry says as much about him as his briefcase. Just the fact that someone is carrying a briefcase tells us quite a bit about him even before a single word is exchanged. He may be a collector of rare antiques or an oil baron. His home may be a chateau. They cannot be brought with you into a business meeting.

Think about the various types of briefcases and the images, correct or not, they convey. The nearly square sample case identifies the carrier as a salesman. The bookbag style case gives the impression of a scholar. A thin leather portfolio suggests its owner needs to carry very little but what he brings is of great importance. A vinyl portfolio says just the opposite. Why would the fact that your case can fall out of an airplane undamaged or be mauled by a gorilla inspire any measure of confidence in you? A fine leather briefcase in a conservative color says all the right things about you, whether you are a new junior executive or established pro. Please, if you possibly can invest in this one item, it will be worth it. A good piece of leather, well constructed, will last for many years and improve with age.

"Watch" Your Style

A gentleman's watch should be plain and simple, made of gold or silver, and preferably does not have a picture of a famous mouse or infamous politician on it. Its band is made of leather, metal, or woven fabrics (gross grain) in a variety of colors. The further away from this you go, the better your chance of spoiling your mature professional look.

There is something distracting about a watch that fires off signal flares and plays the first 16 bars of the "The Star Spangled Banner" to announce the hour. Mini-computer watches have a place, but it's not the board room. Digitals are less formal, and can be less appropriate in the business world.

There are a wide variety of watches that can be perfectly acceptable in any business or dress situation. Names such as Cartier, Rolex, Movado, Concorde, Piaget, and Bulova, to name a few. Most are not only beautiful but also classically elegant.

Class Rings with No Class

There really is no clear-cut time to stop wearing the class ring, a symbol of so many fond memories and not a few broken hearts. But once you've seriously entered into the business world, you should consider retiring it to your jewelry box.

In today's business community it is an unwritten code that you represent your company or your company's product line. Anything that identifies you as a member of some outside group, regardless of how harmless, has the potential of interfering with normal business communications. Selling yourself or your products is tough enough without some unspoken hidden objection hanging around.

Better Belt Behavior

We now turn to that old and venerable friend, your belt. It's such an old friend, in fact, that we tend to take it completely for granted, as if it were invisible. Of course there are other men who do just the opposite; they make an overt display of it (especially the buckle), forcing those around them to focus on a vague area near their belly button. The wrong belt can do as much to keep you from winning as a gaudy tie or poorly cared-for shoes.

Many mistakes you can make with a belt have to do with *selection*. Here are four basic points of selection and use, and solutions to the problems they may engender:

Overly Ornate Buckle

Anything other than a leather (with simple gold or silver buckle) belt is out of place with a traditional business suit. There is a lot to be said for the beautiful works of art available as clasps for sport/casual wear. They can be a terrific way to express a mood or make a statement, but you cannot, must not, try to combine a three-pound piece of turquoise or a replica of the Inca sungod with a business suit.

You may have a good haircut, handsome features, an expensive suit, shirt, and tie. But if you're wearing a belt buckle that's an exact replica of a snub-nose 38-caliber revolver, you can call it quits in the business world.

Brace Yourself!

As clear cut as it may seem, you should always wear a belt when your pants have belt loops. There is one major exception to that dogmatic statement:

Never wear your belt with suspenders (or braces, as they are currently referred to). Both belts and braces serve the same function but they do it in different ways, it's the method of support that's a matter of personal choice. Wear one or the other, but not both. Some folks remove the loops when they have suspender buttons sewn on and some manufacturers don't even include loops if the garment was designed to be worn without a belt. Most often these will be identified by the small tab closure in the front of the pants where the belt buckle would ordinarily be found.

White Plastic Belt with Matching Shoes

Don't do it, plain and simple. It's not desirable or acceptable anywhere. You're asking "Can't a person wear white during the summer and look well dressed?" The answer is yes he can. But not plastic. Consider the time honored and very comfortable white buck popularized decades ago and still around. They are extremely comfortable, reasonably easy to care for, and natural, so they breathe. Combine these with a colored sircingle belt (woven fabric) with white in it and you have the best of both worlds.

Eyeglass Frames: Choosing the Right Ones for You

For some reason, there is a lot of confusion when it comes to selecting the eyeglass frames that look best on you. Sometimes we pay more attention to fashionable or trendy designs or new eyeglass materials that are in vogue, than to the actual materials used in the frames. Are they a color that goes with your eyes and skin tones? Do they go with *the shape of your face*? The most expensive or chic frames on the market will look awful if they don't complement your face.

Study yourself carefully in the mirror, decide which of the face shapes describes you best, and make your selection based on the following proven points:

- **Round:** A round faced man needs to create the illusion of having cheekbones by selecting frames that are straight across the top, angle inward toward the bottom, which is also straight across. Round frames and curved ones should be avoided as they will accentuate the roundness of your face. Stay away from very square styles; they will create too much of a contrast.

Face Shape: Round   *Best Shapes*

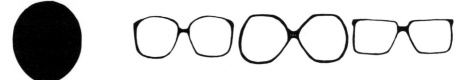

- **Square:** Slightly rounded or curved frames with height on top can modify a square face. Aviator frames often look very good especially if you're young or have stayed in good shape. Your goal is to select a shape that will lengthen the look of your face.

Face Shape: Square   *Best Shapes*

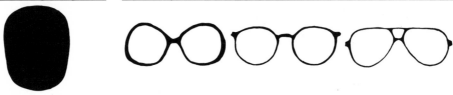

- **Rectangle:** When we refer to this shape we mean long and squarish not short and wide. This shape needs to add some width. A wide, square frame with slightly rounded corners or overall rounded styles seems to create the best look.

Face Shape: Rectangle   *Best Shapes*

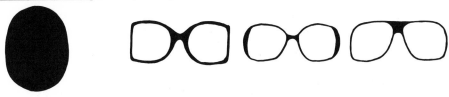

- **Oblong:** The oblong face is long but doesn't have the squareness of the rectangular. Your goal is to add both width and angles. Select slightly wide frames with rounded sides and straight bottoms to add shape. Choose largish glasses with heavier sides.

Face Shape: Oblong   *Best Shapes*

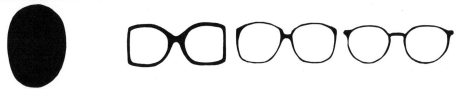

- **Diamond:** The diamond face needs to create the illusion of wider chin and forehead. You need frames with width on top, straight sides, and bottoms that point downward and outward, such as aviator glasses. An oval frame is likely to be a good choice.

Face Shape: Diamond   *Best Shapes*

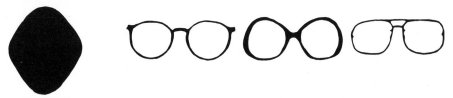

- **Triangle:** This face has a broad forehead and narrow chin. Choose glasses that create balance. The top of the frames shouldn't be heavy and the sides, not wider than your temple. Look for glasses with a curved bottom, similar to the aviator frame. Keep away from square shapes and styles with a heavy bridge.

Face Shape: Triangle   *Best Shapes*

 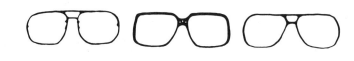

Selecting Style, Materials, and Color

Eyeglass frames that are small in proportion to your face project a natural look, a down-to-earth feel. Proportionate frames—where the amount of glass above and below the eye are nearly equal—are more classic in style. "Aviator" frames or larger frames say "fashion." Women can get by with fashionable frames; for a man, it's much harder. Unless you're in a creative field where expressive attire is acceptable, stick to the functional frames of high quality.

The materials your frames are made of also project various messages about you. Metal frames say "utility." Old-fashioned wire "specs" say "serious." Tortoise-shell or horned rims are "classic." Clear plastic frames are special; they tend to go with just about anything, and, at the same time, they project function and utility. Their versatility is a strong selling point.

When it comes to color, you should key in to your skin tone, hair, and the color of your eyes. Women use pastel, milky, or barely frosted rims to achieve a romantic look. For men, romantic just doesn't work. Stay away from pastels and trendy colors. On men, they look foppish.

Half-glasses are flexible and can go with almost any look, provided the packaging is right. Thin metal half-glasses work to project an expressive look. Heavier metal half-glasses blend with straight hair and fit in with most business uniforms. Tortoise-shells are businesslike.

Silver trims and frames are for cool coloring. Gold is for clear, warm tones. Coppery or bronze-like metals go with a muted warm colors—generally the Autumn palette.

The essential point is to choose frames that harmonize with your natural coloring. It is the surest way to enhance your appearance and maintain the winner's style.

Most men want to be pretty secure.
They don't want to stand out from the crowd.
But they do want to look good.

Richard P. Hamilton
Chairman, CEO, Hartmarx
New York Times Magazine
September 8, 1985

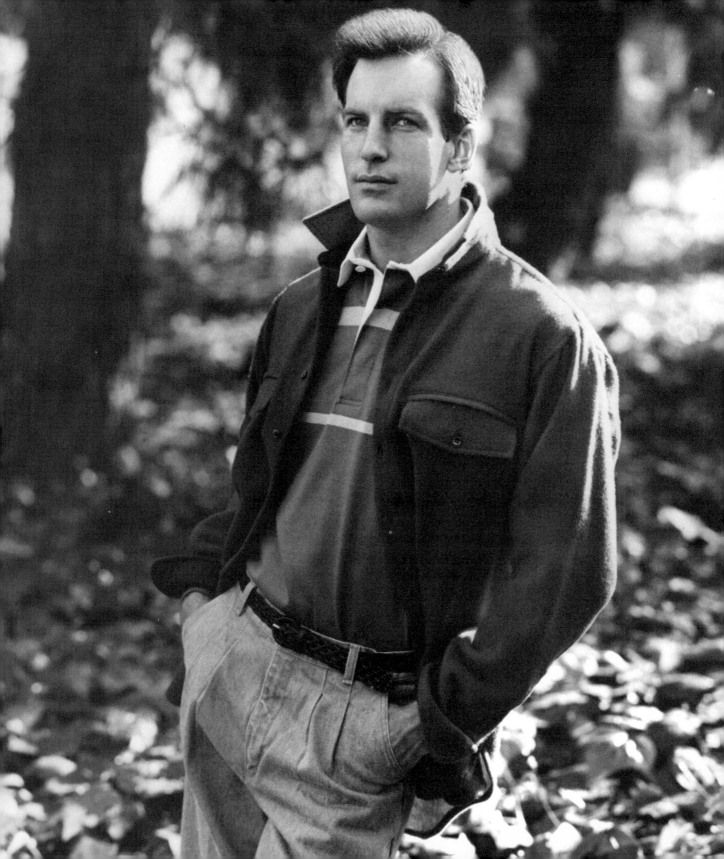

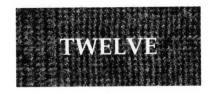

TWELVE

Your Guide to Perfect Grooming

Projecting Your Best

Comedian Billy Crystal, mentioned earlier in this book, uses a very telling and funny line in his "Fernando's Hideaway" routine. Crystal looks at the TV camera for a long moment and tells his viewers, "I know you'd rather look good than feel good, darlings. And you know who you are!"

You may or may not be one of them, but in a business situation looking good can most definitely overcome a multitude of sins. The boss isn't interested in your headache or your aches and pains; he or she wants to fix on a good-looking executive, an executive who realizes that ills come and go, but appearance is forever. Sure, you went overboard a bit at last night's party. But today you've got to close a deal, and you've got to project the kind of poise and confidence and smile that makes the client feel smart doing business with you. It's just good business.

Your suit, tie, shirt, and shoes may be perfect—and that much is expected. Still, there's another side. *Grooming.* It's often the better half of winning someone's respect and trust. A stain on your tie is certainly not in your favor, but the man or woman on the other side of the desk is likely to overlook this small human error if your grooming says better things about you.

Here are some step-by-step guides to make your grooming easier:

Hair Today

It's safe to say that the male "looks revolution" was pulled into the 1980s "by the hair." The decline of the age-old barber shop and the spectacular rise of the men's hairstylist was a precursor of today's preoccupation with the winner's style.

Jon Fultz, one of Washington, D.C.'s hottest hair stylists, works at Robin Weir & Co., Inc., which has made a reputation working with First Lady Nancy Reagan and other Capitol power people. Watching the hair revolution from the inside, Fultz has seen the change of attitude that now allows the average male to have his hair "done" without losing his sense of maleness.

"When you're talking about the corporate environment," Fultz says, "balance is the operative word."

Balance means that the hair is properly cut to match facial structure, that it compliments one's looks as much as any article of clothing or point of grooming. "You should feel as good about your hair as you do your suit," Fultz explains. "The corporate look is 'together'—all together! Everything, including hair, should be clean, right. You shouldn't have to think or fuss about it. Hair should be as natural as anything else about a man. It should have a look that sort of says, 'the hair takes care of itself.' "

Hair Color

Men are coloring their hair these days, which was heresy only a few years ago. The new attitude goes along with today's heightened awareness. Most coloring is aimed at grayness—getting rid of all or part of it. Gray at the temples is still acceptable to men, but premature graying isn't. The prime consideration is the avoidance of the "dyed look." This radical changeover isn't part of the corporate environment, which requires stability from top to bottom. If you are going to color your hair, *do it very slowly.* It should be gradual, so that no one really notices it.

As for doing it yourself, be careful. Many over-the-counter dyes are harsh and damaging. The gray you're trying to get rid of may just fall out if you fail to get the advice of someone, like Jon Fultz, who knows which formulas won't do you in.

A few other tips from the pros:

- If you use a blow dryer, be aware that a high heat setting can play havoc with your scalp and hair, drying both. Keep the heat setting minimal.
- Use a good moisturizer on hair and scalp to reduce any possible damage.
- Men tend to shampoo more than women. Lots of shampooing can also dry your hair and scalp, so use a good conditioner.
- If your scalp is naturally dry, use a shampoo with a light moisturizer in it such as jojoba oil. It's also healthy for thin hair.
- An oily scalp can stand additional drying agents. Again, check with a pro before you cause chemical havoc.
- Normal hair—neither too dry nor oily—needs only a good cleanser. Don't bother with fancy (and fanciful) ingredients.

Hairstyles

Most men are lost when it comes to choosing a hairstyle for themselves. They feel a hairstyle is something they were born with and must maintain for the rest of their lives. Their favorite words when settling into the stylist's chair are, "Same as last time" or "Just a trim, please."

Every good haircut must be styled to the individual. To do that you must pay attention to two key elements: the shape of your face and the type and texture of your hair.

First, determine your face shape:

- **Round Face:** The objective of the cut is to narrow the face. The sleek look of the hair cut evenly in length all around and brushed back from the forehead, with only a partial or no part is preferable. Sideburns, if you choose to wear them, should be on the short side (above the middle of the ear). Brush them back or have the stylist trim them at a very slight angle. Stylist Fultz recommends height on top, and hair a bit longer in the back for a taller look. Prototypes: **John Denver, Ernest Borgnine**

- **Long & Narrow Face:** A rounder style of haircut, with hair a bit fuller on the sides and longer in back, since you need a cut that adds width to your face while maintaining your long neck. Keep sideburns very short (to the top of the cartilage point in the ear). Prototype: **David Hartman**
- **Heart-Shaped or Triangular Face:** The goal, if you have a broad forehead and narrow jaw, is to balance the face; too much hair on top just emphasizes the narrowness of the jaw line. Clip the hair in layers on the top and on the sides. Sideburns should be about one-half-inch below the top of the ear. If the face is narrower at the forehead than at the jaw, a round-type hairstyle, one with a longer, fuller side can help. The idea is to fill in thin temples and deemphasize the jaw line. Prototype: **Fred Astaire**
- **Square Face:** For men this is an excellent face shape. Keep the cut you choose fairly short all around. Since you will look good in just about any cut, discuss with your stylist accentuating one of your finer features: eyes, jaw, or cheekbones. Sideburns should be slightly on the long side (below the cartilage point). Prototype: **Christopher Reeve**
- **Oval Face:** Many people consider this the best of all possible face shapes. You can wear just about any style successfully. Try it short on the sides and long in front, vary the length of your sideburns. Don't feel you have to stick to one look. Talk to your stylist about a style that can be worn conservatively during the day and "let loose" for a night on the town. Prototype: **Jonathan Winters**

Hair Texture

You don't have much freedom when it comes to your hair's texture and type, but here are a few suggestions that may help:

- Thick, curly hair: should always be kept on the short side.
- Fine, straight hair: a short cut will keep it more manageable. If you choose to wear your hair longer, then you must learn to blow dry it properly, using a good natural bristle brush and a styling attachment.
- Thinning hair: should always be cut short, no matter what your face shape is. This makes the hair look fuller. Keep your sideburns short to avoid a lopsided look. As we said earlier, never let your side hair grow long and comb it over the balding area.

Facial Hair

With rare exception, facial hair doesn't work well in business situations. On the other hand, for those willing to be meticulous and who really prefer to wear facial hair, it can be a terrific way to strengthen strong features or minimize weak ones. Depending on your face shape, hair can sometimes be used to create an illusion, much the same way that women use makeup to highlight or disguise certain features. For instance, a medium thick, wide moustache will help broaden a thin face, while a closely trimmed beard, shaped at an angle, will help make a round or wide face look much slimmer. But, if you are one of the many men whose beard is a different color than your hair, you're probably wise to avoid beards and moustaches.

Dandruff

Dandruff, which is usually associated with an excessively oily scalp and white flaking, can often be confused with something as simple as dry scalp. Several friends who thought they would never be able to wear a navy blazer found that frequent washings followed by a good conditioner worked wonders. In certain climates or during the winter months when dry heat is prevalent, a good adjunct to washing and conditioning is to use one of the many hot oil hair treatments available in stores for at-home use, or from your hair stylist or barber. If you choose to try one of the many fine home products, here is an interesting idea: Apply it while taking a leisurely steam or sauna bath.

If the problem *is* dandruff, a qualified dermatologist probably will be your best advisor. While dandruff can't be cured, it can be controlled. And, for those occasions when a small snowfall does occur, a good clothes or lint brush is worth its weight in gold. In a pinch, wrap adhesive tape around your hand with the sticky side out and brush lightly. Keep hands away from your head. No scratching . . . you may cause an avalanche!

Unbalanced Length—Long Back, No Front

When it comes to compensating for lost hair, men can be incredibly creative. However, allowing the hair at the back of the head to grow long is not the way to make others think you have lots of hair. It simply doesn't work! Keeping your hair length proportional to the amount you have will present the best possible look at all times.

If you have lots of hair, wear it as long as is proper for your profession. Lift and lighten it for best results. If, on the other hand, you have precious little hair, take care of it and pamper it. After all, it's all you have!

Too Long

The time for a man's hair to cover his collar in back or completely conceal his ears has passed. The look was a product of the seventies.

Men, being for the most part very conservative, want to stand back and take a wait-and-see position on most matters that have to do with dressing or grooming. The inevitable result is that some men wait until a trend on acceptable fashion has just about ended before they adopt it. Then they walk around for years thinking they really look up-to-date.

Some men think that wearing their hair long somehow compensates for the thinning they wish wasn't happening. It doesn't. It makes them look like they have long, thinning hair.

The current business climate demands a neatly trimmed moderate to short length, keeping all hair where it belongs—on top of the head, not down the back or resting on the shoulders.

Combing Extra-Long Side-Hair Over the Top

This is one of the most difficult ideas for many men to accept; but, allowing the hair on the side of the head to grow to extreme lengths and then combing it in the reverse direction of its natural growth over the top and over to where the other side begins simply doesn't work. It doesn't look like you have a full head of hair, and worst of all is being caught by a gust of wind that blows the hair back to the way it naturally grows. While wearing a hat outdoors works for awhile, you have to take it off, then what? The exact same thing happens when you emerge from your favorite swimming pool, lake, or ocean.

If you've lost the hair, or are in the process of losing it, accept it. It doesn't make you look old or bad. Most men's hairlines recede a bit, so why not blend into the crowd? Toupees or transplants work, if you must. But they have drawbacks: Toupees slip. Transplants hurt.

"Things have certainly changed in this country over the last two decades. Prior to that, being overly concerned with clothes was thought to be highly suspect or unmanly. Today, most men admit to caring about their appearance—their hair, their bodies and their clothes. Of course this has been true in Europe for decades. It is not considered odd for a man to go to his barber two or three times a week to keep up his appearance."

Bill Blass
New York Times Magazine
September 16, 1984

Poorly Groomed Hands

A man's hands are on display virtually every minute of the day. Handing a report to a secretary or colleague, pointing to a column of numbers, shaking hands, and eating lunch are activities that spotlight the very area that most men studiously avoid paying proper attention to each and every day. The reason for this is not because men felt it wasn't important. As a matter of fact, all agreed on the need for clean, well-groomed hands. Of the hundred or so men we talked to, only two had had a professional manicure; one by a girlfriend and the other on orders from his company (his hand was part of a photo to be used in the annual report).

The mystique of the "manicure" seemed to be the culprit behind most men's reluctance. What to expect from a manicurist? First, she will cut and shape your nails to the proper length. Notice that she will cut your nails corner to center, other corner to center and center across tip. Next is a soak. The position of your hands is a little awkward for most guys but it only lasts about five minutes. Then, using an orange stick, usually with cotton over the end, she will gently push back your cuticles. Finally, she will gently buff your nail beds, always going in one direction. Never back and forth. Resist the well-meaning suggestion to have clear polish applied. It is just too shiny. If you want or need a little something, see if a light top coat won't suffice.

All you need is a once-a-month visit to supplement your at-home care; a paltry 20 minutes out of the 43,200 minutes available every month. If you aren't sure that this effort has tangible results, or feel that you do a "good enough" job with your trusty pocket clippers, do a little experiment: try a professional manicurist. The first time you go, have only one hand done and commit to fairly judging the difference. It will be so startling you may not believe your own eyes.

If you're still unsure about visiting a manicurist, the following will help:

Do-It-Yourself Manicure

Some men think of their hands as working objects, as "tools" that are expected to be a bit scuffed and soiled. That's fine if you work out of doors. But in today's corporate environment a workman's hands—which on a true out-doorsman are proud symbols of honest labor—just don't make friends. We may not think it's fair, but it's a fact.

There's another factor at work when it comes to your hands. A lot of men think it's "prissy" to fool with their fingernails. No longer is a manicure just for women. A part of good grooming in a business setting requires well-cared-for hands. You can grouse all you want to, but at some point you've got to accept it and do the best you can. After all, you're not alone and you know that deep down inside a manicure does not a lightweight make!

Your nails grow about a quarter-inch every 10 days. If you don't want to buy a professional manicure you can do it yourself rather easily. Tools needed: emery board (not metal), an orange stick (that's what color it is), a pumice stone (for removing rough spots), a hand lotion (used to soften and mois-turize), a nail buffer (for finishing touches), a small bowl with warm water and a capful of mild dishwashing liquid (for soaking and cleaning).

1. Wash and dry hands thoroughly.
2. Use clipper to shorten the nails (clip from right to center, then left to center, finally across the top to avoid splitting).
3. File briskly with emery board in one direction only. Do one side toward the center and then the other.
4. When your nails are smooth and nicely rounded, place them in the soapy water for about 5 minutes. If you have stains or dirt, now is the time to gently brush them away. This also softens the cuticle and prepares you for the next step.
5. Use an orange stick to gently push the softened cuticles back over the base of the nail. Don't cut!

6. Rub the pumice stone gently around each of your nails, removing dead skin. Put your hands back into the soapy water for a few minutes, then under cool running water. Dry your hands thoroughly and apply a few drops of hand lotion, massaging it into and around the nails. Finally, in a brisk back and forth motion, buff your nails to a soft gleam. Don't get them too shiny.

Skin Care

For some reason, men don't think much about their skin. They should, since it's the most visible part of the body. It needs cleansing, exercise, rest, and proper nutrition just like the rest of you. Like a winning smile, your skin mirrors your health and way of life. Here are some basic tips that will help you look fit and healthy:

1. Always cleanse your skin with lukewarm water. Using extremes of temperature can be harmful. Very hot water, for instance, opens the pores dramatically and brings subcutaneous oils to the surface. Years of this kind of action can increase oiliness, enlarge pores, and permanently stretch out their elasticity. Cold water will roughen your skin as much as repeated exposure to arctic winds.
2. Invest in "smart water"—either distilled or natural spring water. You can drink it and wash with it, making it good inside and out. These waters have fewer chemicals and salts, and your skin truly appreciates this touch of kindness.
3. Stimulate your face. Give it a mini-massage. Stand in front of the mirror and make faces at yourself. It's a form of exercise that tones the facial muscles and heightens color. All forms of exercise will help promote skin tone and a healthy complexion, but don't forget to make those funny faces a few times a week. It needs only a few minutes to bring excellent, long-lasting results.
4. Feed your face. But feed it the proper foods. If you're taking in a lot of cell-withering sodium chloride (ordinary table salt) you'll develop wrinkles at an early age. Caffeine in excess will do the same, and an excess of refined grains and sugars can produce spots. The best nutrients are rich in Vitamin A and Vitamin E. Honey, used externally, will help

regulate moisture content. Proteins, enzymes, minerals, collagen, RNA, elastin—there's a vast assortment of helpmates out there. Go to your local health food store and ask questions. The results can be startling.

5. Think prevention. If you're a smoker, you should be aware of a 1971 study by Dr. Harry W. Daniell which relates smoking to crow's feet around the eyes. Once you hit the 40 to 49 age bracket, he says, you are likely to appear as wrinkled as a non-smoker 20 years your senior! Overexposure to the sun is another wrinkler—or worse. Recent studies indicate substantial increases in skin cancer among those who just can't seem to get enough tanning. Take the sun in small doses and moisturize with products containing PABA or benzehenone.

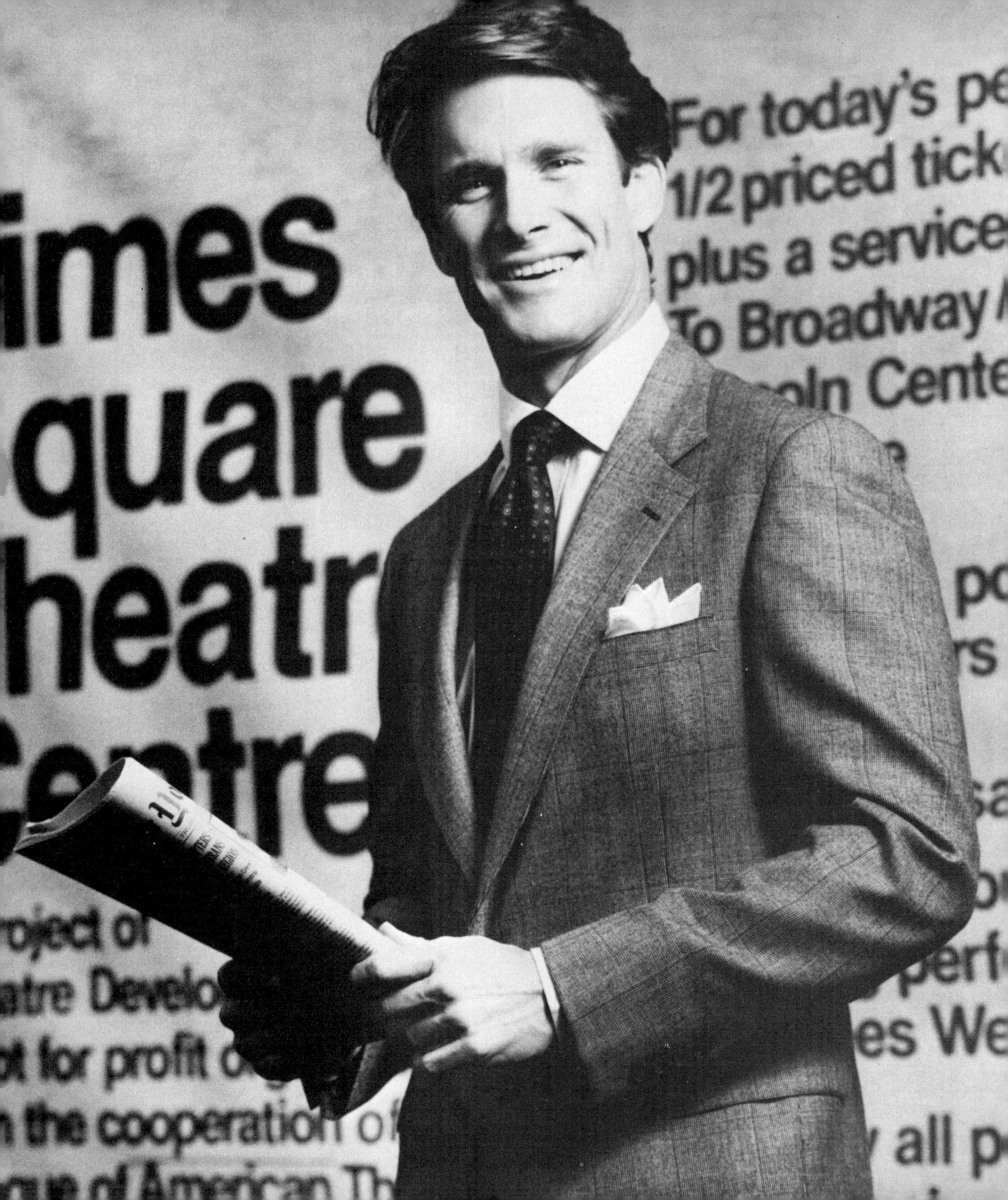

imes
quare
heatr
For today's pe
1/2 priced tick
plus a service
To Broadway
oln Cente
roject of
atre Develo
ot for profit
n the cooperation o
es We
all p

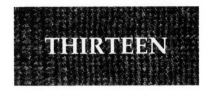

Polishing Your Image

Do You Qualify?

"Look at your business card. Does it look crisp, clean, together? Surely *you* should look as good as the card you're handing to a potential client."

The quote comes from an "image consultant." It's her business to make people look great—and she does. She knows color, fabrics, tailoring, hair, skin care—just about everything cosmetic you can think of.

The image consultant points out that, in the above example of the business card, it was designed and printed by professionals. Her job is similar because she, too, designs a look and sends it out into the world where it can be seen and judged by all.

Does it work?

"Definitely," says Bob Adler, a New York designer of mens' clothing. "The image people are even having an impact on the major manufacturers."

Today thousands of men are turning to the pros. And not only the individual; whole corporations are also taking advantage of the geometrically expanding image-maker industry. What they gain is very simple: executives who project a winner's style—one good enough to eventually show up in an earnings report.

Men are relative newcomers to a market that's been booming for women in the past five years. Until recently, men felt uncomfortable at a hairstylist salon and few would ever dream of putting their images into the hands of trained color consultants. All this has changed, and men have followed the women into a quest for practical, no-nonsense advice from the pros. To their delight, it *works*!

Shopping for a Consultant

What is an image consultant exactly? How does he—in this case mostly she—operate?

It's hard to give exact definitions, but there are general guidelines for defining various consultants available to you today:

- An "image consultant" looks at the whole person. In addition to dress, attention is given to the way you project in public, the way you "come off" in the presence of peers. Color is used extensively in matters of wardrobe, and there is a healthy dose of finishing school etiquette that helps you feel more confident in social situations.
- A "color consultant" is a little more specialized than the image-maker, though both aim at the same finished product. The color consultant is expert in matters of physical coloration—they match you with your best looking wardrobe options. They provide a good deal of advice on how and where to shop for quality clothing, where to get a good hairstyle. In the end, they hope for a poised, good-looking customer, who now has enough information to make his or her own decisions about what works best.
- The "lifestyle" consultant is, in a way, a bit psychoanalytical. This group goes beyond wardrobe and looks. It aims to help you change a whole way of life—or at least certain major portions of living. The lifestyler gets into personal issues, and though it's a great concept, the lifestyler may be a bit too complex for the average corporate executive.

Telephone books in every major city in the United States list several columns of image and other related consultancy services. But finding the right consultant for you isn't as easy as picking up a telephone and making a call to a listing in the directory. Before making that call you need to do some initial homework, including a certain amount of soul-searching.

Dianne Neidigk, head of Full Service Total Image Consulting, in Tomball, Texas, says that most men arrive at her office first having learned to people-watch and second having formed some strong opinions about what they can gain from her.

"Before a man uses a consultant," she says, "he should have a pretty good idea of what he wants out of life generally. It isn't enough just to say you want to look good. You need a *reason*. When I know what a man is aiming at, I can help him get it more efficiently and achieve exactly what he needs."

Men from all walks of life find themselves in Neidigk's office. One of her first customers was a maintenance man in the Texas public school system. Like most men who go to a consultant for the first time, he felt slightly uncomfortable, maybe even silly. "But he knew what he wanted," Neidigk recalls. "He had noticed how women used color and how it helped their appearance. He wanted to know how it worked. In the end, it improved his feelings about himself and raised his confidence level tremendously."

Besides the total look, men use consultants to find out about quality clothing and where to buy it. They want information on tailoring, fabrics, styles, grooming. The result, Neidigk says, is that men gain information from a consultant to confidently make choices on their own. The consultant may go shopping with a client, but hopefully (and typically) the client is on his own.

What kinds of specific advice are men seeking?

"First of all," Neidigk says, "they want hard, fast answers. They're not interested in complicated color theories."

A lot of men seek help in the area of appropriate dress in a given situation. It isn't unusual to find men being intimidated and confused when faced with all the options in a clothing store—what to buy for when. And for what occasion?

"It's a contagious thing," Neidigk explains. "Men look around and see all the trends—the hairstyles, the new colors. They begin to see that they may need a little guidance out there, just as all of us do."

To make the most of it, she emphasizes, the clients have to "like themselves today." If they are interested in improving their appearance, "they need the self-confidence to follow through on it."

Some men are looking for substantial makeovers, but most are after strategic information. Salesmen, for example, use consultants to obtain an "image of the day"—the right look at the proper time. A really good salesman knows that his dress for a small town client isn't the same as it is in the big city. "It makes perfect sense," Neidigk says. "You don't show up at a small rural hardware store in your 'power suit.' "

Using Your Good Instincts

Harold Nelson, vice president and general manager of Neiman-Marcus in Washington, D.C., says men should look upon image consultants the same way they view any other kind of learning experience.

"I've been playing golf for 15 years," he says, "and never took a lesson. Then one day I did, and my game improved vastly after six holes. It's the same with your image. You can think of it like learning how to order the right wine or negotiate for a house. It's all learned behavior."

Nelson advocates shopping around. "Go out and try different consultants. Get second opinions. Look for someone with whom you agree on a gut level, because not every consultant is right for you personally."

The question men have to answer, he says, is this: Is something wrong with me, and, if so, is it holding me back? If your answer is yes, seek professional input.

"Once you find someone," Nelson continues, "realize that you're going to hear criticism. If you can't take it, you're in trouble."

It's best, he adds, to develop a good one-on-one relationship. And it's up to the consultant to prove the case of whatever is best for you. "Men are creatures of habit," he says. "Changes are tough. And you shouldn't have to make dramatic changes. Look for fine-tuning—not radical makeovers. This happens too much. A consultant should build on what is best, not tear everything down and start over . . ."

He says it's important to keep in mind that a consultant, by virtue of the business they're in, will find problems to solve. It's a little like going to a mechanic and asking if your car needs working on. The answer most of the time will be yes, because that's what the mechanic is in business for. There is a misconception about men and style—or rather their alleged ineptness when it comes to style, Nelson explains. "There are men who do the right things but who lack confidence and need reinforcement. That's why it's important for a consultant to build on the basic structure. After all, if it's not broken, why fix it?"

Men must also ask themselves: is there a need for change, or is the change only an experiment? Nelson wisely warns that thinking that a change in appearance automatically takes care of other problems in your life or career is foolhardy. But looking right—and being appropriate for any situation—covers a multitude of sins.

"Let me give you a very simple example," he says. "You want to feel good about yourself, right? Sure. So you go to a baseball game in 90-degree heat in a three-piece suit because you see the owner of the team wearing a three-piece suit. The owner looks okay. But you are out of place, inappropriate, and you feel dumb. That's because the team owner is appropriate for his role, but you as a fan are not."

What to Look For

How do you know which consultant is best for you?

The best way is to ask a lot of questions. Ask them who they trained with, and for how long. Who have they worked with? Have they done corporate consulting? If so, that's a definite plus.

Prices for this service are reasonable. A typical one-hour session with a consultant (at the office) costs about $40 to $60. For $50, you can find consultants who will spend an hour shopping with you. Very well-known consultants charge hundreds of dollars an hour for similar services. For about $500 worth of consulting, you could learn about your colors, your wardrobe, basic grooming, and how to put it all together in a smashing way.

Consultants often hold seminars, which are advertised on television and in the newspapers. Sometimes these group sessions are more productive than individual treatment. Groups provide immediate feedback, and it's easier for a lot of people to interact with others about common goals. For about $100 you can have a consultant make an individual video for you, and in a group situation you can buy the same thing for a lot less.

Does it really work?

"You bet," Dianne Neidigk exclaims. "Men are the biggest supporters of consultants once they see how much it can do for them."

Winning Tips on Consultant Selection

1. Know what you want before you get there.
2. Have a clear idea of how you'll put the information to work for you.
3. Shop around. Not all consultants are right for you. Find the one you're most comfortable with.
4. Be wary of a consultant who wants to do a complete makeover on you. You should build on your strong point; keep the basic man intact.
5. Gain confidence. Have a consultant go shopping with you if you feel you can't go it alone. But aim for making all your own decisions.

6. Be aware of your "look of the day." The right look at the right moment. You may be comfortable with nine out of ten situations—but don't hesitate to seek advice on that one area of concern.

7. Think of the consultant's service as a "lesson," a class you might audit at a local university. You're there to learn.

8. Take advantage of group situations. They're inexpensive and social. The feedback is excellent.

9. If changing something about you really feels *wrong*—seek a second opinion.

10. Think about making a video. It may cost $100 or so, but it might well be the best investment in your overall appearance you've ever made.

"I firmly believe that what gives other people a sense of what and who you are is the way you are dressed. It is the first impression. I can't think of a man who, whether in business or leisure, does not want to project authority."

Bill Blass
New York Times Magazine
September 16, 1984

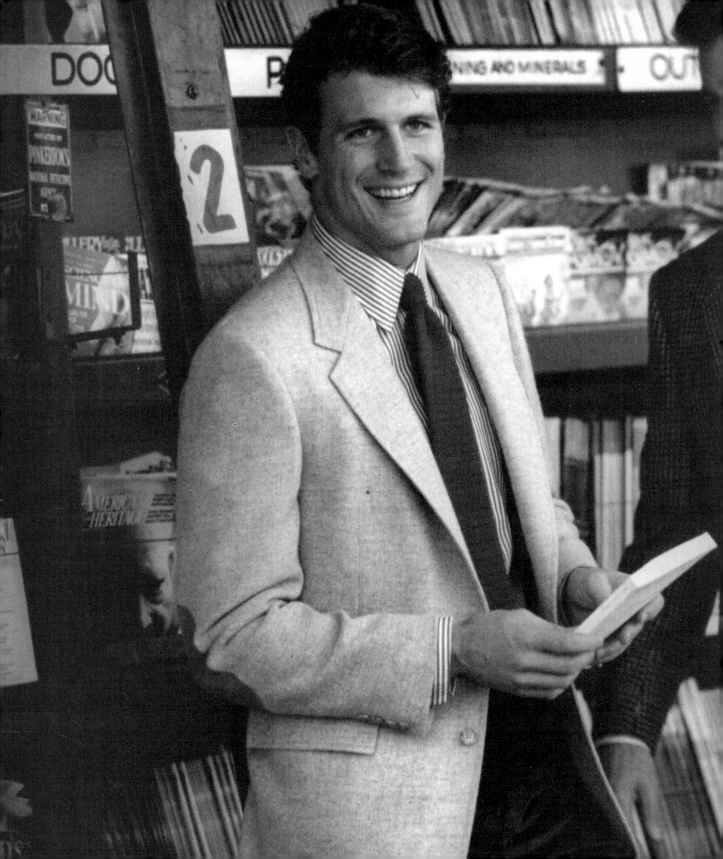

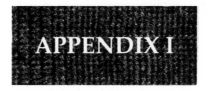
APPENDIX I

Male Maintenance Manual

At Loose Ends?

The very same man who treats his automobile as if it were his most cherished possession can sometimes be the same gentleman who treats his clothing as if it were an alien invader from outer space. This isn't always the case—but too often it is. Could it be that men know more about the complex innards of their BMWs than they do about sewing on a button? Painfully, the answer appears to be yes!

There are all sorts of reasons put forth to explain this phenomenon. Sociologists point to American's "love affair" with their automobiles. Psychologists say men gravitate toward gadgets and leave the buttons to mom. Chauvinists of the male variety speak gruffly of "woman's work," while their female counterparts insist that men don't have the tactile abilities required to properly handle needle and thread.

In the end, all sides may have valid points to make. But it doesn't solve the problem, and, meanwhile, men keep showing up at the office literally at loose ends. If you're one of these unfortunate souls, that's a shame. Chances are you won't get much in the way of sympathy from your male colleagues, and the women who want to "mother" you only reinforce your lack of skills.

So, let it end here! What follows are a lot of little tips that will go a long way toward putting your loose ends back in shape, where they belong. They add up to yet another component of the winner's style.

Sewing on a Button

Buttons are always popping off of garments at the most inconvenient time—while preparing for a major meeting with the top brass, or a thousand miles from home in a hotel room 30 minutes before a presentation to a very important client. Unless you travel with a personal valet, there will be times when having this basic repair skill will prove invaluable.

When you come across a loose button, try to figure out where it came from, as it's always easier to sew on a button as soon as possible after it falls off. If this isn't possible, have a box or bag set aside where orphan buttons can wait until the garment-sans-button is located. If the button is lost and replacements must be purchased, here is some technical information you'll need:

Button size is measured across the diameter in "lines," 40 lines to the inch. Most of the buttons used on a suit (the sleeves, lining pocket, vest front, trouser fly, and back pocket) are 24 line buttons. The jacket front is usually a 30 line button. Horn or dull bone buttons are your best bet with a classic suit of fine material. Mother of pearl or synthetic buttons are most common on shirts. Today many fine manufacturers sew on an extra button to the tail of their shirt fronts in the event emergency repair is necessary.

Once you have the button, you'll need a one-and-a-half-inch-long needle with a medium-sized eye. Needles are divided into sharps and betweens. Betweens are generally shorter and stronger. Sharps are medium to long in length. In both categories the needle sizes are numbered. The higher the number, the shorter and thinner the needle. A #7 sharp should take care of most repairs. Choose a color of thread that matches either the thread on the other buttons or that closely matches the color of the garment. Mercerized cotton thread #0 or #00, or size A silk thread is suitable for most sewing jobs.

To thread the needle, cut off about a foot of thread, wet one end to help create a point. Push the thread through the needle's eye and pull it through. Tie the two ends together. If you have trouble with this, a needle threader helps.

Position the button on the garment and, starting on the wrong side of the fabric, push the needle through a hole in the button. Push the needle back through another hole in the button. Sew in an X-pattern if it's a four hole button; make paralleled stitches in a two-holer. After about six stitches, wrap the thread around the button stalk, push the needle back through the fabric and secure with a few small stitches across the back of the new button. Cut off any excess thread and, violá, you're done.

Missing Buttons

I am not an unsympathetic person. I really feel badly for the guy who puts on his last clean shirt, goes to his car and while turning his head to back out, pops a button. Usually, it is the collar button. No amount of tie tightening will conceal it. The spread of your collar will be affected and people will know that your top button isn't buttoned. They won't know if your neck is too fat to allow your shirt to close, you've just lost the button, or you're a slob who just doesn't care.

If you use a commercial laundry, they will very often replace a missing button for you as part of the service. If you do not, try to check for loose or cracked buttons before you toss your shirt into the laundry basket. "A stitch in time saves nine," applies here, too. Many hotels provide miniature sewing kits consisting of a few buttons, a needle, and variety of threads to help their guests who find themselves in need. Such a kit should be part of every man's travel kit and also a part of his "junk drawer" at the office. If the idea of sewing is alien to you, at least try to be creative until you get your shirts back from the cleaners, out of the wash, or whatever. I remember meeting with the president of a cosmetics company. In the course of the afternoon we removed our jackets. He was missing a button on his left sleeve cuff. The cuff was being held together by a safety pin. If he had a little more style, flash or "je ne sais quois" he should have pulled or cut off the button on his other cuff and pinned them both. People may have thought it was a new style of cuff link.

Stain Removal

It never hurts for your next door neighbor to be a professional dry cleaner. In the event that he is off sunning himself in St. Tropez, however, you should have a few household chemicals handy for emergencies. You should be able to deal with most problems if you have access to the following:

- Liquid dishwashing detergent
- Clear, non-fragranced ammonia
- Peroxide bleach (be careful to test on a non-visible part of the clothing, it could stain)
- White table vinegar
- A commercial enzyme presoak
- A liquid grease solvent

There are a few very common "solutions" that are used for a variety of cleaning situations. They are:

- Enzyme solution—except in special circumstances which will be noted, it is a quart of warm water with one tablespoon of presoak detergent solution—one-half teaspoon of detergent *diluted* in one quart of warm water.
- Ammonia/detergent solution—same as the detergent solution with the addition of one tablespoon of ammonia.
- Vinegar/detergent solution—same as the detergent solution with one tablespoon of vinegar added.

Food or Perspiration Stains

Through his necktie a man has the opportunity to express some small part of his inner self without going too far from what most of us consider conventional attire. It would be a shame to mar this statement by walking around with sweat or spaghetti sauce all over it.

The painfully obvious solution is to have your ties properly cleaned and avoid accidents. It is, at times, impossible to prevent something from landing on your tie while on its way to your mouth. When the inevitable does happen, I suggest two ways to deal with this problem: keep an extra shirt and tie in a box in your car or office (depending on where your normal work day finds you).

If, for some reason, this idea is not possible and you must face the prospect of being seen by others with a synopsis of your lunch visible on your tie, you may as well point out that you've had an accident. It has been my experience that most people are very sympathetic and will actually pay closer attention to your face or presentation when they are given half a chance!

Removing Stains in Washable Garments

You will have much more success removing soil from your washable garments than your nonwashables. The following list is a mini-bible:

Alcohol, Coffee, Tea, Soda—gently daub with ordinary tap water; if this doesn't do, go to a detergent solution. If you have a particularly stubborn stain then go to a detergent and ammonia mixture. If after all of this there is any remaining stain, use a little peroxide. Beer responds very well to soaking for one half hour in an enzyme solution.

Ballpoint pen ink—daub with solvent. Rub with soap and wash if the stain is still there. Sometimes spraying hairspray on the spot, allowing it to dry brushing it off will do the trick, too.

Blood—ordinary tap water (always cold) should be tried first. If this doesn't work, try the detergent and ammonia solution. A drop or two of peroxide should help clear up any final traces.

Catsup/Chocolate—daub with dry solvent first, let dry. If the stain remains, try a detergent solution and after that a detergent/ammonia solution if necessary.

Cosmetics (including lipstick)—daub with cleaning solvent.

Fruit juice—sponge the area immediately with cold water. Daub with white vinegar if you don't discover the stain until it has dried. If necessary, presoak and wash.

Grass stains—daub with solvent and let dry. Next, soak in a detergent and vinegar solution. Use peroxide for particularly stubborn stains.

Mustard—scrape off excess mustard carefully and daub with a cleaning solvent or powder. When stain persists, daub with detergent/vinegar solution.

Pencil—rub gently along the grain of the fabric with a soft eraser. If this doesn't remove the marks, wet the stain with detergent, add a few drops of ammonia if necessary.

Alcohol—soak immediately with club soda and rinse in water.

Removing Stains in Nonwashable Garments

- **Alcohol, Coffee, Tea, Soda**—daub with vinegar and rinse.
- **Ballpoint pen ink**—daub with solvent. If the spot remains, send it to the dry cleaner.
- **Blood**—a few drops of ammonia should do the job.
- **Catsup/Chocolate**—wet the stain with a solution of one-half teaspoon of presoak and a half-cup of warm water. Let it stand for a bit before you rinse with cool water.
- **Cosmetics** (lipstick)—if a quick application of cleaning solvent doesn't clear it up, it must go to the dry cleaner.
- **Fruit juice**—try cold tap water first, then white vinegar if the stain has dried. If this doesn't work, then you have no choice but to send it to a dry cleaner.
- **Grass stain**—sponge on a cleaning fluid and let it dry, or you can try a cleaning powder.
- **Mustard**—scrape off any excess mustard carefully (you don't want to spread it around) and daub with cleaning solvent or powder. Where the stain persists, daub with detergent and vinegar solution.

Ironing a Shirt

In the best of all possible worlds you would never discover that your favorite all cotton shirt didn't go to the laundry or your permanent pressed shirt loses its permanence. When you do or when it has, you only need access to water, an iron, a towel, a sheet or pillowcase, and a flat surface.

For the most part, shirts are easier to iron when damp, not after they are completely dry. If they have dried, use a pump-spray mister to dampen the shirt as you iron. Or, put your shirts in a plastic bag in the vegetable crisper section of the refrigerator for a few hours. The combination of the cold fabric and hot iron will produce a crisp, well-pressed shirt.

Now, start ironing with the yoke of the shirt and go from there to the collar, doing the inside first and then go on to the outside, pulling as tautly as you can while ironing.

Next do the back, the sleeves, and then the cuffs. Iron the front last. Begin on the button side of the shirt, iron around not over the buttons. There is usually an indented groove around the toe of the iron which will allow you to go around and under the buttons. When you get to the button hole side be especially careful when ironing the placket—that is where the buttonholes are. The entire front should be ironed from the collar to the tail.

Do-It-Yourself Eyeglass Repairs

The vast majority of men have not discovered that eyewear can be used for more than correcting vision problems. Instead of considering eyewear as a piece of jewelry or an accessory, which can be used to their advantage in complimenting the skin tone and face shape, they view them as an appliance to help them see.

And, as with all appliances, men think that a little tape, a paperclip or a yard of bailing wire can fix anything as good as new. All that these short-cut fixes do is establish a fellow as someone who is clever enough to save $2.87, (which is what you'd have to pay to have a professional do the repair), at the cost of looking like a nerd.

If you travel a great deal, it's a good idea to pack an extra pair of eyeglasses with your toiletries. That way, if you should accidentally sit on your glasses in your hotel room, you won't be forced to make that million-dollar presentation with a paperclip hanging down next to your temple or a roll of white adhesive tape on the bridge of your nose. If this is a recurring problem, solve it once and for all by buying a kit containing the proper replacement parts and the tools to make the repairs yourself.

Protecting Your Investment Or
How to Decode the Labels in Your Clothes

The labels sewn inside your clothing are there as a guide to proper care and feeding of the rather substantial investment you've made in a winner's wardrobe. Unfortunately, some of these sewn-in instructions, especially those from foreign countries, seem written for experts in Sanscrit. One day we'll have uniform, easy-to-understand instructions sewn into all our clothing, but until that fine day arrives we have no choice but to decipher the often cryptic codes the various mens' clothing manufacturers have handed to us.

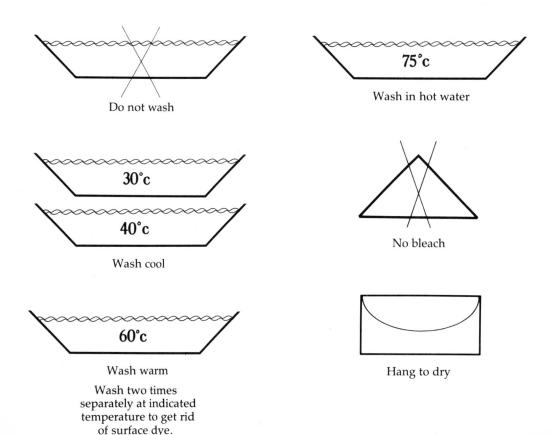

Do not wash

75°c
Wash in hot water

30°c
40°c
Wash cool

No bleach

60°c
Wash warm

Wash two times
separately at indicated
temperature to get rid
of surface dye.

Hang to dry

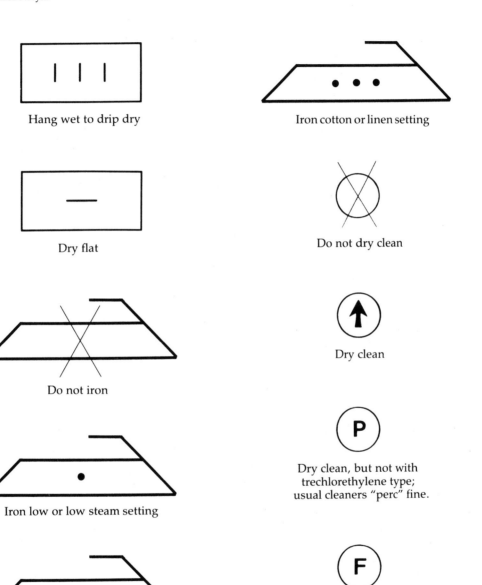

Hang wet to drip dry

Iron cotton or linen setting

Dry flat

Do not dry clean

Do not iron

Dry clean

Iron low or low steam setting

Dry clean, but not with trechlorethylene type; usual cleaners "perc" fine.

Iron medium setting

Dry clean only with petroleum or flourocarbon solvents.

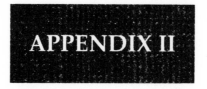

Winner's Resource Guide

The Winner's Resource Guide is an overview of the best known manufacturers in the country. Included are listings for *suit/sport coats* and *shirts*.

The following information is provided for each manufacturer:

Brand name: What name appears on the label. Names of the parent companies are noted in parentheses.

Address: Usually the main showroom.

Distribution: Whether or not their products are nationally available.

Type of stores: Where to look for this brand.

Type of fit: See chapter three for definitions and more information.

Author's comments:

Price range:

Special note: If you are a consumer, and you don't see a favorite brand listed, or you are a manufacturer who would like to be listed, please write to me, Ken Karpinski, *c/o* Acropolis Books Ltd., 2400 17th Street, N.W., Washington, D.C. 20009-9964.

Suit/Sport Coat Manufacturers

GIORGIO ARMANI
650 5th Avenue, New York, NY 10019

National distribution: ☒ *Yes* ☐ *No*   Type of stores: ☐ *Department* ☐ *Speciality* ☒ *Both*

Phone numbers; *Showroom:* **(212) 265-2760**   *Cust. Service:* _____

Type of fit: **European – 7" drop**

Author's comments: **Very sophisticated styling and fabrics, most models ventless. The couture line is approx 20% higher.**

Price range: **$700 – $950**

BILL BLASS (PBM)
1290 6th Avenue, New York, NY 10104

National distribution: ☒ *Yes* ☐ *No*   Type of stores: ☐ *Department* ☐ *Speciality* ☒ *Both*

Phone numbers; *Showroom:* **(212) 581-8270**   *Cust. Service:* **(212) 581-8270**

Type of fit: **Modified American – 6" drop**

Author's comments: **Known for its taste level and fabrications. Well priced, with mass appeal. Represents a good value.**

Price range: **$250 – $300**

BROOKS BROTHERS
346 Madison Avenue, New York, NY 10017

National distribution: ☒ *Yes* ☐ *No*   Type of stores: ☐ *Department* ☒ *Speciality* ☐ *Both*

Phone numbers; Showroom: __(212) 682-8800__ *Cust. Service:* _____

Type of fit: Full cut - 5" drop
"346" line - 6" drop / Brooksgate Line - 7" drop

Author's comments: Known for the integrity of the garment, and consistency of the product. It enjoys a tradition of fine quality and workmanship. A classic in the best sense of the word.
Price range: __$300 - $500__

BURBERRY
9 East 57th St., New York, NY 10020

National distribution: ☒ *Yes* ☐ *No*   Type of stores: ☐ *Department* ☐ *Speciality* ☒ *Both*

Phone numbers; Showroom: __(212) 581-6510__ *Cust. Service:* _____

Type of fit: Updated Modified American - True English

Author's comments: Quality, value, & exclusive English piece goods for the upscale male.
Price range: __Approx $395__

CRICKETEER—JOS. & FEISS (PHILLIPS, VAN HEUSEN
290 Avenue of the Americas, Suite 1914, New York, NY 10104

National distribution: ☒ *Yes* ☐ *No*   Type of stores: ☐ *Department* ☐ *Speciality* ☒ *Both*

Phone numbers; Showroom: __(212) 581-6750__ *Cust. Service:* _____

Type of fit: Traditional American 6" drop
Cricket Club 7" drop

Author's comments: High quality at a reasonable price. Consistent fit which will serve you well over a long life. Everyone from new college graduate to company president can be suited.
Price range: __$260 - $285__

COUNTRY BRITCHES
1290 Avenue of the Americas, New York, NY 10019

National distribution: ☐ Yes ☐ No   Type of stores: ☐ Department ☒ Speciality ☐ Both

Phone numbers; Showroom: __(212) 581-6750__   Cust. Service: _____

Type of fit: Updated Traditional

Author's comments: Refined taste level — a very high-quality product. Elegant, understated approach to fashion. Exceptional value.

Price range: _____ $350 - $425 _____

HART, SCHAFFNER, MARX (HARTMARX)
1290 Avenue of the Americas, New York, NY 10104

National distribution: ☒ Yes ☐ No   Type of stores: ☐ Department ☒ Speciality ☐ Both

Phone numbers; Showroom: __(212) 397-3620__   Cust. Service: __(800) FAS·HION__

Type of fit: Full cut- 6" drop
regatta - traditional american
ambassador European

Author's comments: Famous for its quality and consistency of fit. The label has become a sign of quality and value. It is hard to go wrong with this garment.

Price range: _____ $375 — $400 _____

HASPEL (PALM BEACH)
1290 Avenue of the Americas, New York, NY 10104

National distribution: ☒ Yes ☐ No   Type of stores: ☐ Department ☐ Speciality ☒ Both

Phone numbers; Showroom: __(212) 247-5771__   Cust. Service: _____

Type of fit: Modified American — 6" drop

Author's comments: A classic, almost a legend for this type of garment. Best light-weight, fully-tailored, wash & wear suit in American. Should be a part of most men's warm-weather wardrobe.

Price range: _____ $130 — $200 _____

HICKEY FREEMAN (HARTMARX)

1290 Avenue of the Americas, New York, NY 10104

National distribution: ☒ *Yes* ☐ *No*   Type of stores: ☐ *Department* ☒ *Speciality* ☐ *Both*

Phone numbers; Showroom: **(212) 397-2530**   *Cust. Service:* **(716) 467-7240**

Type of fit: **Modified American — 6" drop**

Author's comments: **Hand-crafted garment made of the finest imported fabrics available. The comfort, ease, fit and feel distinguish this garment from most mass-produced garments. Their motto: Try A Hickey-Freeman on for size.**

Price range: **$600 - $800**

PALM BEACH

1290 Avenue of the Americas, New York, NY 10104

National distribution: ☒ *Yes* ☐ *No*   Type of stores: ☐ *Department* ☐ *Speciality* ☒ *Both*

Phone numbers; Showroom: **(212) 581-7520**   *Cust. Service:* _____

Type of fit: **Gentleman's Fit — 6" drop**
            Signature Line — 7" drop

Author's comments: **Manufactured in the U.S.A., cut and produced for the American male. Well made at an excellent price. Available in a wide variety of fabrics and colors.**

Price range: **$180 - $250**

PIERRE CARDIN (INTERCONTINENTAL BRANDED APPAREL, INC.)

888 7th Avenue, 15th Floor, New York, NY 10106

National distribution: ☒ *Yes* ☐ *No*   Type of stores: ☐ *Department* ☐ *Speciality* ☒ *Both*

Phone numbers; Showroom: **(212) 397-2810**   *Cust. Service:* _____

Type of fit: **European   7" drop**
            "Pour Homme"   6" drop

Author's comments: **First designer to design for the American man. Good variety of fabrics and colors. Fine attention to detail.**

Price range: **$250 - $400**

POLO by RALPH LAUREN
40 West 55th Street, New York, NY 10019

National distribution: ☒ Yes ☐ No   Type of stores: ☐ Department ☐ Speciality ☒ Both

Phone numbers; Showroom: (212) 581-8434   *Cust. Service:* _____

Type of fit:

Author's comments: *Tailored of fine fabric, styled for american male. conservative yet sophiscated.*

Price range: _____ $600 - $850 _____

SOUTHWICK
10 West 55th Street, 4th Floor, New York, NY 10019

National distribution: ☒ Yes ☐ No   Type of stores: ☐ Department ☐ Speciality ☒ Both

Phone numbers; Showroom: (212) 581-8434   *Cust. Service:* _____

Type of fit: *Modified American 6" drop*

Author's comments: *Famous for its soft-shoulder elegance. Excellent craftsmenship, fabrication, and attention to detail. Conservative styling.*

Price range: _____ $350 - $600 _____

STANLEY BLACKER
1290 Avenue of the Americas, Suite 1529, New York, NY 10104

National distribution: ☒ Yes ☐ No   Type of stores: ☐ Department ☐ Speciality ☒ Both

Phone numbers; Showroom: (212) 246-3232   *Cust. Service:* _____

Type of fit: *Basic American 6" drop*

Author's comments: *Fine durable product made in the U.S.A. Finest fabrics at a fair price. Updated clothing which will not be outdated in years to come.*

Price range: _____ $250 - $275 _____

VAN JULIAN
17 West 54th Street, New York, NY 10019
National distribution: ☒ *Yes* ☐ *No*   Type of stores: ☐ *Department* ☐ *Speciality* ☒ *Both*
Phone numbers; Showroom: **(212) 582-1572**   *Cust. Service:* **(212) 582-1572**
Type of fit: Updated Modified Traditional 6" drop

Author's comments: Extremely well-priced, with strong intrinsic value. Extra attention is paid to the details.
Price range: _____ $189⁹⁵ - $250 _____

JOHN WEITZ
600 Madison Avenue, New York, NY 10022
National distribution: ☒ *Yes* ☐ *No*   Type of stores: ☒ *Department* ☐ *Speciality* ☐ *Both*
Phone numbers; Showroom: **(212) 752-8860**   *Cust. Service:* _____
Type of fit: Modified American 6" drop

Author's comments: Geared toward the business and professional man. Made in the U.S.A. Good quality fabrics and workmanship.
Price range: _____ $180 - $250 _____

Y.S.L. (BIDERMANN)
1271 Avenue of the Americas, New York, NY 10020
National distribution: ☒ *Yes* ☐ *No*   Type of stores: ☐ *Department* ☐ *Speciality* ☒ *Both*
Phone numbers; Showroom: **(212) 541-6750**   *Cust. Service:* _____
Type of fit: European - 7" drop

Author's comments: Well known name in Designer clothing. Sophisticated fabrications and colors.
Price range: _____ $225 - $400 _____

Shirt Manufacturers

ALEXANDER JULIAN
8 West 40th Street, New York, NY 10018
National distribution: ☒ *Yes* ☐ *No*   Type of stores: ☐ *Department* ☐ *Speciality* ☒ *Both*
Phone numbers; Showroom: **(212) 382-3700**   *Cust. Service:* _____
Type of fit:
          Traditional

Author's comments:

Price range: _____ **$30 - $60 (depending on fabrication)**

ARROW
530 Fifth Avenue, New York, NY 10036
National distribution: ☒ *Yes* ☐ *No*   Type of stores: ☐ *Department* ☐ *Speciality* ☒ *Both*
Phone numbers; Showroom: **(212) 930-2900** _ *Cust. Service:* _____
Type of fit: *Traditional*
          Fitted
Author's comments:

Price range: _____ **$30 - $60 (depending on fabrication)**

CHAPS (WARNACO)
261 Madison Avenue, New York, NY 10016
National distribution: ☒ *Yes* ☐ *No*   Type of stores: ☐ *Department* ☐ *Speciality* ☒ *Both*

Phone numbers; Showroom: **(212) 490-0800**   *Cust. Service:* _____
Type of fit:
Traditional

Author's comments:

Price range: _$30-$60 (depending on fabrication)_

CHRISTIAN DIOR (WARNACO)
261 Madison Avenue, New York, NY 10016
National distribution: ☒ *Yes* ☐ *No*   Type of stores: ☐ *Department* ☐ *Speciality* ☒ *Both*

Phone numbers; Showroom: **(212) 599-2280**   *Cust. Service:* _____
Type of fit:
Fitted

Author's comments:

Price range: _$30 - $60 (depending on fabrication)_

EAGLE (PALM BEACH)
1290 Avenue of the Americas, New York, NY 10104
National distribution: ☒ *Yes* ☐ *No*   Type of stores: ☐ *Department* ☐ *Speciality* ☒ *Both*

Phone numbers; Showroom: **(212) 245-5600**   *Cust. Service:* _____
Type of fit:
Traditional

Author's comments:

Price range: _$30 - $60 (depending on fabrication)_

GANT (PALM BEACH)
1290 Avenue of the Americas, New York, NY 10104
National distribution: ☒ *Yes* ☐ *No*   Type of stores: ☐ *Department* ☐ *Speciality* ☒ *Both*

Phone numbers; Showroom: **(212) 581 - 7520**   *Cust. Service:* _____
Type of fit:
          Full-Cut

Author's comments:

Price range: ____$30 - $60 (depending on fabrication)____

GITMAN BROTHERS
39 West 55th Street, New York, NY 10019
National distribution: ☒ *Yes* ☐ *No*   Type of stores: ☐ *Department* ☒ *Speciality* ☐ *Both*

Phone numbers; Showroom: **(212) 266 - 2821**   *Cust. Service:* _____
Type of fit:
          Traditional

Author's comments:

Price range: ____$30 - $60 (depending on fabrication)____

HATHAWAY (WARNACO)
90 Park Avenue, New York, NY 10016
National distribution: ☒ *Yes* ☐ *No*   Type of stores: ☐ *Department* ☐ *Speciality* ☒ *Both*

Phone numbers; Showroom: **(212) 697 - 5566**   *Cust. Service:* _____
Type of fit:
          Full - cut

Author's comments:

Price range: ____$30 - $60 (depending on fabrication)____

PIERRE CARDIN (PALM BEACH)
53 East 57th Street, New York, NY 10022
National distribution: ☒ *Yes* ☐ *No*   Type of stores: ☐ *Department* ☐ *Speciality* ☒ *Both*

Phone numbers;   Showroom: **(212) 245-5600**   *Cust. Service:* _____
Type of fit:

      Fitted

Author's comments:

Price range: _____

VAN HEUSEN (PHILLIPS, VAN HEUSEN)
1296 Avenue of the Americas, New York, NY 10104
National distribution: ☒ *Yes* ☐ *No*   Type of stores: ☐ *Department* ☐ *Speciality* ☒ *Both*

Phone numbers;   Showroom: **(212) 541-5200**   *Cust. Service:* _____
Type of fit:

      Fitted & Traditional

Author's comments:

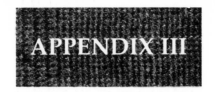

Glossary

Batiste: A sheer, lightweight weave that is good for warm weather.

Bedford Cord: A relatively heavy fabric with a raised cord (similar to corduroy), running lengthwise. Differs from corduroy in that it is made of wool and is not stiff.

Boat Shoe: A casual, moccasin-style loafer with a heavy lace running around the top, tying at the instep. It usually has a sturdy crepe or rubber sole.

Braces: Another name for suspenders, they are used to hold up pants.

Broadcloth: A fabric that is closely woven with a very light, crosswise rib. It can be identified by its smoother, tightly woven finish, giving it a dressy look.

Button-down Collar: A collar held down at the points by buttons.

Camel Hair: The wool-like underhair of the camel which is lustrous and extremely soft. It is used either by itself or combined with wool. The natural colors range from light tan to brownish-black. It is used generally in outercoats and sports jackets.

Cashmere: A fine grade of wool from the long-haired Kashmir goat. It is a soft, elegant fabric with a slightly fuzzy surface.

Chest Piece: A coarse fabric that fits between the outer fabric and the lining to help a suit coat hold its shape.

Cheviot: A twill simlar to serge, but with a slightly round, napped surface. It is more suitable for business than a smoother, dressier suiting.

Club: A tie pattern where heraldic devices or sports symbols are diagonally repeated on a solid background.

Collar Bar: A gold or silver-colored bar that attaches to the points of the collar and keeps it in place.

Collar Stays: The plastic strips that fit inside the thin groove sewn into the underside of a collar point.

Cook Shield: Made by Warren K. Cook, it replaces the jacket sleeve button with an enameled "button" with the family crest on it.

Cordovan: Although often confused with leather, it describes a dark black-red color and a subcutaneous cartilage found in the hindmost parts of a horse.

Corduroy: A ribbed fabric of cotton, polyester, rayon, or blends. It may have wide or narrow wales and is usually stiff.

Cream Polish: Used on leather shoes, it feeds fine leather and keeps it supple.

Double-breasted: A type of cut of a jacket characterized by a double thickness of material across the breast and having a double row of buttons.

Ectomorph: A body type characterized by being slim, tall, and having long, linear muscles on the arms and legs.

Endomorph: A body type characterized by a round body, often described as pear-shaped.

End-on-end: A fabric woven from alternating white and colored fibers, creating a grainy, almost checkered look.

Epaulet: A shoulder ornament such as on a military uniform.

European Cut: A close-fitting suit with padded shoulders, waist emphasis, and high armholes.

Fitted: A close-fitting shirt ideal on a trim silhouette.

Foulard: A lightweight silk tie fabric with a very fine twill weave. It has a small, evenly-spaced, geometric pattern on a solid background.

Full: A comfortable, loose-fitting shirt.

Full-lined: An additional layer added on a suit jacket, it provides extra protection against the cold, helps the jacket slide on and off easily, and also helps the jacket to lay smoothly on the shoulders.

Gabardine: A firm, tightly woven fabric of wool or cotton (or cotton and polyester blend) with a fine diagonal ribbing. It comes in many weights and makes a durable suit, jacket, or slacks.

Gap-osis: A condition that exists when a man's vest does not come down far enough to cover his belt line.

Gig Line: The line formed by a man's shirt button placket, the edge of his belt buckle, and his trouser fly.

Glen Plaid (*crisp*): A subtle plaid that needs to keep a crisp line to maintain the straight overall effect.

Glen Plaid (*flannel*): A subtle plaid that will soften the effect of the straight line because of the flannel.

Goodyear Welt: The most expensive, as well as most familiar, method of attaching the sole of a shoe to the uppers. It has a grooved effect that runs around the sole.

Gucci Loafer: A dressy loafer with a piece of distinguishing hardware across the instep.

Half-lined: An additional layer added to summer suits. It helps the jacket to slide on and off easily and to lay smoothly on the shoulders.

Harris Tweed: Woolens handwoven on the islands of the Outer Hebrides off the coast of Scotland.

Herringbone: A zigzag woven pattern suggesting the skeleton of a fish. Rows of chevron stripes are woven into contrasting or close colors to form this pattern.

Hopsack: A coarse and loosely woven fabric with a basketweave effect. It is used for suits, jackets, and slacks.

Houndstooth Check: A broken twill, four-pointed star check, somewhat reminiscent of the fangs of a dog.

Ivy League Cut: A suit in which the jacket has natural shoulders, hangs straight, and has a center vent. The slacks are plain and hang straight.

Linen: A fine textured, strong cloth made of flax. Because it sags and wrinkles so easily, it is often blended with man-made fibers for longer-lasting shape.

Melton: An overcoating with all-wool warp and weft; the face is napped carefully, raising the nap straight, to show the weave clearly.

Mesomorph: A body type characterized by natural proportions and a good muscle structure.

Natural Shoulder: Also called the sack suit, it has little or no padding, low-cut armholes, and little waist emphasis.

Notched Lapel: A fairly wide V-shaped opening at the outside edge of the seam between the collar and the lapel.

Overplaid: A double plaid on which the weave or, more often, the color effect, is arranged in blocks of the same of different sizes, one over the other.

Oxford Cloth: A cotton fabric with a small basketweave surface, used for shirts. It is slightly less formal than broadcloth.

Paisley: A pattern used for ties that can be both elegant or sporty depending on the colors.

Peaked Lapel: A lapel of a jacket or coat that comes to a point at the outer edge and points upward.

Penny Loafer: A basic loafer with a cut-out over the instep.

Photogray Lenses: A particular type of lens for glasses which is able to adjust to the available light.

Pima Cotton: A fine grade of cotton made from long, smooth fibers.

Pinpoint: This shirt fabric is woven with two different color threads which, gives a very subtle blending of a pin dot.

Pinpoint Oxford Cloth: A weave that is more tightly woven than oxford, but much softer than broadcloth.

Pinstripe: A very fine stripe, usually less than one-sixteenth of an inch.

Piping: A contrasting colored fabric that is sewn into the edges and lapel of a jacket.

Pocket Square: A silk handkerchief worn in the breast pocket.

Polyester: A man-made fabric that can be spun, patterned, and woven in such a way as to resemble wool. It can also be combined with natural fibers to create a more soft, resilient, and practical blend.

Poplin: A strong medium-weight, plain-woven fabric with fine crosswise ribs, made of cotton, silk, wool, blend, or man-made fabrics.

Raglan Sleeve: A sleeve made of one piece continuing to the collar.

Reprocessed Wool: Yarn made from wool that has been woven, knitted, or felted into a wool product that without ever having been used has been returned to a fibrous state.

Rise: The distance between the base of the crotch of a pair of pants and the waistband.

Saxony: A general term for the finest quality woolen made of staple, botany wools of superior felting power. It may be stocked-dyed, piece-dyed, or yarn-dyed.

Sea Island: A weave even more sheer than batiste that is very expensive.

Seasonal Color Theory: A theory using undertone, depth, and clarity to relate a person to a season. This season is then applied to describe a person's coloring and the range of colors that flatter that person.

Seersucker: A light weight cotton fabric with crinkled stripes made by weaving some warp threads slack, and others tight.

Serge: A twill weave with the diagonal prominent on both sides of the cloth.

Shantung: A plain silk weave characterized by a rough, nubbed surface caused by knots and slubs in the yarn.

Sharkskin: A smooth-finished, clear-faced, twill-weave fabric made of one color crossed with white. It is used in worsted for suits and coats, and in silk for neckwear.

Shetland: A wool gotten from sheep raised in the Shetland Isles of Scotland. It is usually woven with a raised finish and soft hand. It is most commonly associated with sweaters.

Silk: A soft, fine, shiny fabric made from fibers produced by silkworms as they form their cocoons. It is resilient and wrinkle-resistant when woven into a fabric.

Single-breasted: A type of jacket cut characterized by the overlapping of the front just enough to be fastened by a single row of buttons.

Skirt: The bottom of a suit jacket that covers a man's rear end.

Slub: A soft lump or thick irregular place in yarn.

Solid: A single colored tie in silk, wool, cotton, or a blend of fibers.

Spread Collar: A narrow, wide spread collar that needs to be worn with a large knotted tie.

Striped: Sometimes called rep stripe, regimental, or school tie, it is a striped tie in silk, wool, cotton, or a blend of fibers.

Suede: Leather of which the flesh side has been buffed to a smooth finish.

Tab Collar: The shirt collar is held together by the use of tabs.

Tassle Loafer: A type of loafer that has leather tassles (sometimes metal tipped) that hang over the instep.

Tattersall: A checked pattern in one or two colors on a light background.

Tie Tack: A tack, usually with an ornate head, used to hold the tie in place.

Top Stitching: A zigzag stitching on the outside of a suit. It is usually the designer's "signature."

Traditional: Often referred to as a gentleman's cut, the shirt is cut fuller across the chest and not fitted at the waist.

Trench Coat: A double-breasted overcoat with a wrap-around belt. It was designed after military trench coats worn in World War I.

Tweed: A rough surfaced wool fabric of two or more colors, usually soft and flexible.

Twill: A closely woven worsted with pronounced slanted lines in texture. It is easy to care for and press.

Updated American: Also called Modified American, it is a two-button suit that has lightly padded shoulders, slight tapering at the waist, and is higher in the armholes.

Vent: The opening usually in the back of a suit. It can also be double-vented or sometimes referred to as side-vented.

Vicuna: The wool of the vicuna, a llama-like animal of the Andes, the finest fiber classified as wool. It can be identified by its reddish-brown color, pronounced silk luster, and exceptionally soft hand; however, it wears badly and is not recommended.

Virgin Wool: According to the Wool Products Labeling Act of 1939, virgin wool, also called new wool, is "wool that has never been used, or reclaimed from any spun, woven, knitted, felted, or manufacturer, or used product." The term is no guarantee of quality, because any grade of wool can be called virgin wool.

Warp: The threads running lengthwise in fabric.

Wax Polish: Used on leather shoes, it brings up a shine and is somewhat water resistant.

Weft: The threads running horizontally in fabric.

Whipcord: Usually a bold warp twill, with about a 63 degree angle and a clear finish that emphasizes the diagonal cord or twill. It is a very sturdy, service-able fabric.

Windsor Knot: A formal, symmetrical, and extremely stylish tie knot done using a double wrap technique.

Wing Tip: A shoe with the tip in the shape of the spread wing of a bird, with perforated seams and toe-cap design.

Wool: The fleece of sheep which can be woven into many different forms.

Worsted: A very smooth-surfaced wool fabric woven of worsted (twisted) yarn spun from the hard "tops" of raw wool. It is generally more expensive than woolens.

INDEX

A

Academy of Fashion and Image,
  28, 55
Accessories
  belts, 13, 120, 121
  braces, 121
  briefcases, 30, 119
  pens, 118
  pockets, 118
  rings, 120
  suspenders, 121
  wallets, 115
  watches, 119
Adler, Bob, 139
Ali, Mohammed, 18
Always In Style, 14, 61
Athletic Cut, 45

B

Beauty for All Seasons, 57
Belts, 13, 120, 121
Bogart, Humphrey, 25
Boots, 111

Bowties, 95
Boxer shorts, 56
Braces, 121
Briefcases, 30, 119
Briefs, 55
Brokaw, Tom, 25
Bush, George, 24
Buttons, 68, 148, 149

C

Carole Mosbacher and
  Associates, 61
Carson, Johnny, 25
Case studies, 37, 41
Chest piece, 65
Collar, 67
Color,
  cool, 97
  eyeglass frames, 124
  hair, 128
  questions, 102
  shoes, 103
  socks, 103
  warm, 97

Color Concepts, 58
Color Me Beautiful, 60, 96
Color Planner
  Autumn, 100
  Spring, 101
  Summer, 99
  Winter, 98
Color Theory,
  benefits of, 103
  seasonal, 96
Connors, Jimmy, 26
Corporate Image Checklist, 28
Crystal, Billy, 17, 127
Cuffs, 80

D

Dandruff, 131
Davis, Karen, 59
Dickerson, Mike, 56

E

Erikson, rubye, 60
European cut, 45
Eyeglasses
  checklist, 28
  color, 124
  do-it-yourself repairs, 153
  materials, 124
  shapes, 122-124
  style, 124

F

Fabric, 75
Face shapes, 122-124, 129, 130
Fixx, Jim, 26
Full Lining, 48
Full Service Total Image
    Consulting, 141
Fultz, Jon, 128

G

Gap-osis, 68
Grooming, 127

H

Hagler, Marvelous Marvin, 19, 26
Hair
  color, 128
  dandruff, 131
  facial, 28, 131
  length, 132, 133
  style, 28, 129-130
  stylists, 128
  texture, 130
  tips, 129
Hoehndorf, Norma, 56
Hogan, Hulk, 27

I

Illusion dressing, 58
Image consultants,
    advice, 28, 55, 56, 58, 60, 63,
        141, 144
    shopping for, 140, 144
    types of, 140
Image consulting firms, 28, 55, 56,
        58, 60, 61, 141, 144
Image Reflection for Body and
    wardrobe, 61
Ironing, 152

J

Jackets, 29, *see also: suits*
Jackson, Joyce, 56
Jewelry, 15
Johnson, Don, 19, 23

K

Karr, Norman, 21, 44
Koppel, Ted, 25

L

Lapel width, 65
Leisure wear, 55

M

Maintenance
    buttons, missing, 149
    buttons, sewing, 148
    ironing, 152
    laundry care labels, foreign, 154
    stain removal, 150
Manicure
    do-it-yourself, 135
    professional, 134
Man-made fibers, 69
McEnroe, John, 26
McMahon, Jim, 27
Mosbacher, Carole, 61

N

Natural Shoulder, 44
Neidigk, Dianne, 141, 144
Nelson, Harold, 142

O

Oakland, Virginia, 61
O'Neill, Thomas "Tip", 24
One on One Fashion Consulting,
        61

P

Palmer, Arnold, 58
P.A. Principle, 58
Pens, 118
P.I.C.C., 56
Pocket squares,
    checklist, 30
    folding, 116

Q

Quinn, Anthony, 24

R

Reagan, Ronald, 19, 24
Rings, 120
Robinson, Joanne Hull, 61

S

Scott, George C., 23
Shirts
    checklist, 29
    collar, 71
    contrast stitching, 77
    fabric, 75
    ironing, 152
    non-dress, 74
    patterns, 75
    short sleeved, 77
    too tight, 75

Shoes
    boots, 111
    checklist, 31
    dress, 111
    gunboat style, 110
    how-to-buy, 108
    quality, 107
    repair, 111
    shoe shine, 109
    unpolished, 110
Shoeshine, 109
Size chart (European), 51
Skin care, 136
Socks, 113
Sports coats, see suits
Stain removal, 150
Stockman, David, 23
Style
    adventurous, 57
    aristocratic, 57
    conservative, 57
    corporate image checklist, 28
    eyeglass frames, 122
    geographic, 28, 60
    hair, 28, 129
    rustic, 57
Suits
    athletic cut, 45
    buttons, 68
    buying, 43
    chestpiece, 65
    collar, 67
    color, 98-101
    European cut, 45
    fit, 44, 49, 52, 64
    full lining, 48
    lapels, 65

man-made fibers, 69
natural shoulder, 44
pattern, 66
pinstripes, 66
piping, 64
styles, 44
three piece, 48
two piece, 48
updated/traditional American
    cut, 45, 46
Suspenders, 121

T

Third Piece Dressing, 61
Thompson, Bobbie Jean, 61
Ties
    bowties, 95
    checklist, 30
    knit, 93
    length, 88, 93, 94
    patterns, 86, 89
    tacks, 94
    too wide, 92
    tying troubles, 87
Tie tacks, 94
Trench coats, 31
Trousers
    checklist, 30
    crease, 81
    cuffs, 80
    fit, 82
    pockets, 80
    waist size, 81

U

Ultimate Image, 56
Underwear
    boxer shorts, 56
    briefs, 55
Updated/Traditional American
    cut, 45, 46

V

Vests
    Gap-osis, 68
Virginia Oakland and
    Associations, 61

W

Wallets, 115
Watches, 31, 119
Watson, Thomas, Sr., 18
Weinberger, Casper, 25
York, Brenda, 28, 55

Always in Style
How to Make Fashion Work for You
Line, Proportion & Color
by Doris Pooser

- ***75,000 hardcovers sold—now in quality paperback!***

The revolutionary book on individual body shapes, style, and color is now available to more persons than ever! *Always in Style* offers new style and color options that will expand the range of your fashion personality, including exclusive color "flow" charts that enable you to wear colors from another season! First, you'll learn your own "body line" to determine those styles that go best with your proportions. Then, you'll find out how to identify your skin's undertone, intensity, and clarity that will lead you to colors from another season!

   Always in Style will give you the confidence to choose the best style, to make your own spectacular fashion statement!

   Doris Pooser heads up the fashion consulting firm Accolade, Inc., and 125 Always in Style consultants.

ISBN 87491-823-5/$9.95   quality paper/Beauty
Publication Date: November, 1986
196 pages, 8 × 9, illustrated throughout, 40 full color photographs (including 6 seasonal color flow charts), 60 illustrations.

Color Me Beautiful *Updated*!
Discover Your Natural Beauty through Color

by Carole Jackson

Now with millions convinced that color can work miracles in your life—here is the brand-new updated *Color Me Beautiful.*

The "basics" are the same...*Color Me Beautiful* is "the no-diet instant beauty book." The secret is still in the color seasons. For, just as nature is divided into four distinct seasons, you have a unique skin tone and coloring in tune with either *Winter...Summer ...Spring...Fall.*

Carole Jackson tells you how to discover your "season" and how to use the 30 sensational colors in your "seasonal palette" to make your wardrobe, hair color, makeup, and accessories just right.

This updated edition contains vital new information on a new way to tell your "season," wardrobe planning and clothing personality, and lovely new illustrations!

ISBN 87491-756-5/$14.95 hardcover/Beauty
212 pages, 24 page color section, b/w illus.